THIS IS AN ADVANCE UNCORRECTED PROOF BOUND FOR YOUR REVIEWING CONVENIENCE.

In quoting from this book for reviews or any other purpose, it is essential that the final printed book be referred to, since the author may make changes on this proof before the book goes to press.

Advance Praise for *The Pet Healer Project: Stories of the Healing Bond Between Humans and Animals*

"One of the most extraordinary books I've ever had the pleasure of reading. It is full of positive stories about animal lovers working miracles within the animal and human kingdoms. One astonishing tale after another recounts the steps of recovery, rediscovery, transformation and healing. Every page lifts your spirit. No stranger to the metaphysical healing movement, I was nodding my agreement after each paragraph. The book is a remarkable read, well written and enthralling. I am inspired and moved by it. I wish every person on earth could read it and understand the powerful, spiritual, life-altering bond we have with animals. There were many sentences I loved from this author, but one in particular stood out in my heart. "For me, it's really about the spirit and compassion, and that underneath our differences of species, we're really the same. True healing is about healing our spirit and remembering that we are all one. And that's really what our lives are all about isn't it? Remembering that we are all one."

KAC YOUNG PHD, AUTHOR, THE (SUPPOSEDLY) ENLIGHTENED PERSON'S GUIDE TO RAISING A DOG. HUBBLE & HATTIE. 2017

"A few years ago, when bringing my Collie back from a devastating paralysis, it would have been wonderful to add healers, along with doctors, to her recovery team. Sandy explores these dedicated people in the Pet Healer Project, and skillfully opens up an exploration of new understanding and connection of the bonds between our pets and ourselves.

Beautifully written and passionately expressed."

TOM MOORE, THEATRE AND FILM DIRECTOR AND ANIMAL ADVOCATE

"This brilliant work marks the emergence from a time where pets are "treated like animals." Now, for most of us, our pets are family. As family members, they receive the love and nurture they need to grow and heal. Yet as anyone who has been nurtured and healed by the warmth of a bedside dog can tell you, healing is much more than medicine. *The Pet Healer Project* explores the power of that connection; bringing us deep inside the mind, spirit, and practices of the pet healers that exemplify this.

Perhaps we're one step closer to a day where we focus on healing not only our pets with our minds and spirits, but also our planet."

MARK ROBINSON, FOUNDER OF WALKIN' WHEELS BY HANDICAPPEDPETS.COM

"After producing many films around the world involving the animal kingdom, I was excited to read about these distinguished healers, teachers and veterinarians who offer new and innovative insights on how to best take care of animals. Providing a wealth of options, both mainstream and alternative, we learn of different approaches to healing, rehabilitation and communication and, most importantly, how to ensure that our beloved pets lead a happy and healthy life!"

MASHA NORDBYE, AWARD-WINNING DOCUMENTARY PRODUCER/ DIRECTOR AND AUTHOR.

Sandy Johnson

November 2017

The Pet Healer Project

Stories of the Healing Bond
Between Humans and Animals

the *Pet* Healer Project

Stories of the Healing Bond Between Humans and Animals

SANDY JOHNSON

TOP READS PUBLISHING, INC

Vista, California

First Edition

ISBN-10: 0-9964860-5-4
ISBN-13: 978-0-9964860-5-7

Library of Congress Control Number: 2017949353

The Pet Healer Project: Stories of the Healing Bond Between Humans and Animals is published by: Top Reads Publishing, Inc., 1035 E. Vista Way, Suite 205, Vista, CA, 92084-4213 USA

For information please direct emails to: topreadspublishing@gmail.com or visit the website: www.TopReadsPublishing.com

Cover design: Teri Rider
Book layout and typography: Teri Rider & Associates

Printed in the United States of America

Please Note:
The information given in this book is not intended as a substitute for professional veterinary or medical advice. Many of the healing techniques should be considered as therapies to be used alongside the care, treatment and advice provided by a veterinary doctor, and a veterinary doctor must always be consulted for any concerns or problems whatsoever with a pet or other animal. Neither the author nor the publisher can be held responsible for any loss or claim arising out of the use or misuse of the suggestions made in this book nor the failure to take professional veterinary advice.

For Charley

CONTENTS

INTRODUCTION | *1*

CHARLEY'S ANGEL | *5*

MARY DEBONO | *Me and My Best Friend* | *13*

KATHLEEN PRASAD | *The Light at Brookhaven* | *23*

CAROL KOMITOR | *A Voice for All God's Creatures* | *33*

KAREN BECKER | *The Shaman's Apprentice* | *43*

LESLIE GALLAGHER | *Water Babies* | *57*

ELIZABETH WHITER | *Pegasus* | *69*

ALLEN MARK SCHOEN, DVM, MS, PH.D. (HON.) | *The Middle Path* | *77*

CINDY BRODY | *CinergE* | *89*

JAMES FRENCH | *The Trust Technique* | *97*

EILEEN HAWORTH | *The Doolittles of Topanga Canyon* | *107*

MARGRIT COATES | *An Urgent Message* | *115*

ANTHONY GEORGE | *West Meets East* | *123*

ANNA BREYTENBACH | *A Walk in Anna's World* | *135*

MARC CHING | *Undercover Angel* | *151*

EPILOGUE | *163*

ABOUT THE AUTHOR | *165*

ACKNOWLEDGEMENTS | *167*

WHERE TO FIND OUR HEALERS | *169*

INTRODUCTION

The world of healers has always fascinated me. Knowing that just outside the borders of our perceived reality is a whole other universe of mystery and magic and unlimited possibilities has always called to me.

A few years ago, when I was researching one of my books on healers, I attended a conference at UCLA. Scientists and doctors shared the stage with energy healers to discuss the differences in their approaches to health and healing. The issue on that day was the placebo effect. Placebo, from the Latin *I shall please*, points to the brain's role in medical treatment; whether it's the doctor the patient wants to please or the patient's belief system the doctor wants to reinforce or the medicine itself. Sugar pill or protocol, the placebo response has played an important role in medicine for more than two hundred years.

One of the speakers, an oncologist, told the well-documented story of "Mr. Wright," a cancer patient suffering from late-stage lymphatic cancer. Wright made a practice of reading medical journals; one day he read that a certain horse serum was shown in clinical trials to be effective on cancer. Begging and pleading, he got the doctor to include him in the trial. Within weeks, Wright's tumors began to melt away and he was feeling great. Ten days later, Wright was discharged from his "death bed." A few months later, a story appeared in the medical journal stating that recent studies proved the serum to be totally ineffective. Almost immediately

Wright had a relapse, the tumors returned, and in a matter of months he was dead.

I was particularly moved by this story. I had always wondered about the placebo effect even while writing about the many successes of various healers. In 1996, when I interviewed the Dalai Lama for *The Book of Tibetan Elders,* I put the question to him. "Yes," he answered, "the placebo is the mind's own physician."

Next, a veterinarian from Germany presented slides showing X-rays of a nine-month-old puppy that had been hit by a car. The dog's hind leg was badly broken, the tibia and fibula (shin bones) were completely separated from the femur (thigh bone). The vet informed the devastated family that this kind of break would never heal; if they wanted to save the puppy's life the leg would have to be amputated. As it happened, the puppy's owner was a healer. Refusing to accept either option, the family took the puppy home. Immediately the healer began Reiki treatments, a form of energy healing developed in 1922 by a Japanese Buddhist.

The vet presented the next series of slides. One week later, the puppy's leg was beginning to knit. The next slide, an X-ray taken one month later, showed that the bones had healed completely! Pointing to the last slide on the screen she said, "Here is a photo of the puppy running and playing. Of course, this puppy had no belief or non-belief in the healer's ability to heal, entirely ruling out the question of the placebo effect."

Remove the placebo effect and what we're left with is the very existence of energy healing itself. The proof it seems is in the puppy.

There must be more people who specialize in working with animals, I thought. Calling on my network from my previous books on healers, I packed my virtual bag and laptop and took off, hopscotching (electronically) across the country and even across the pond to England to find them. And since my travels were virtual, Charley (my nine-year-old Brussels Griffon) could remain firmly planted on my lap. I followed wherever the trail led me, and along the way I met the most extraordinarily gifted, highly educated, and accomplished people whose lives are dedicated to the health and well-being of our four-legged companions. Not the garden-variety psychic healers popular among today's New Agers, many of these pioneers in the field of complementary health hold advanced degrees in various sciences. Their love and compassion for animals inspires in each of us a more profound sense of humanity.

These everyday angels walk among us, hardly noticeable except when they're harnessing their power and directing it onto some ailing or injured four-legged or winged or crawling creature. I came across some demons, too, that made me want to look away, but then I came across an undercover angel whose heroic rescues got my attention.

The Pet Healer Project is a collection of their amazing and often miraculous stories.

CHARLEY'S ANGEL

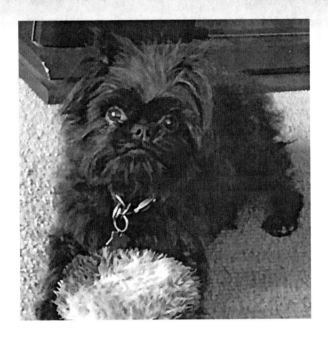

The morning in early May 2007, I woke up with a bad case of puppy fever. Anyone who's ever come down with this condition knows how serious it can be. A puppy was such a bad idea at that particular time in my life for so many reasons that I stopped counting them and called my friend Alex instead. Alex had worked in a veterinary clinic many years ago, and remained a devoted animal lover; and like me, she lives alone. And like me, hates the silence of a house without a pet. "Here's why I shouldn't do this," I said to her, thinking about my recent recovery from cancer treatments. "I mean, what if?"

But then, in the same breath I told her about a Maltese breeder I had heard about thirty-five miles out of L.A. (Tashi Delek, my beloved Maltese had passed away three years before).

"Well, let's go!" she shouted. Puppy fever is also contagious.

There were eight little balls of fluff, one cuter than the other. And none of them Tashi. If I was still comparing every puppy I saw to Tashi maybe it was still too soon. I was about to give up when suddenly a different one, this one jet black came streaking into the room chasing a ball more than half its size. First the puppy rolled it along the floor then pounced on the ball, hard enough to bounce it in the air, and chased it again. The Maltese pups did not move an inch, they just watched.

"What is that?" I asked.

The woman explained she was a Brussels Griffon, left with her by another breeder who was going out of business. She reminded us that it was a Brussels, a brown one, that was in a recent Jack Nicholson movie. We did remember; how could we forget that smart, comical, monkey-faced dog?

The little black puppy had managed to hold the ball still, presumably while deciding on her next move, then, abandoning the ball, she ran over to us and came to a stop right in front of me and looked up at me. Tail wagging furiously, her big black eyes looking directly into mine, she dared me to say no.

I named her Charley.

What I loved about Charley, what drew me to her, was her single-mindedness, her fierce determination to live life. I didn't know it at the time (or maybe I did) but over the coming years I would learn my greatest lesson about the body's ability to heal from her.

Meantime, that same determination had turned into a battle of wills in which the victor is always the one with the cute little monkey-face and the big dark eyes. She was impossible to train. I had just started on a new book and needed to meet a deadline, and Charley never seemed to tire. One minute she was playing with one of her toys, the next she was leaping onto the couch then flying off it and zooming to the door demanding to go out. She liked meeting other dogs and testing her rank in the neighborhood pecking order.

She also liked to shop. Our local pet store keeps a variety of bones in open bins a few inches off the floor giving dogs an opportunity to sniff them out; Charley chose one of the large, heavy ones that she could tame into submission. At the cash register I noticed a card: Chris's Critter Sitter, Dog Walking, Puppy Training, Day Care Services. I asked about it. "She's great," he said. "I use her myself." I looked at Charley, Charley looked back at me. What d'you think? Charley blinked, shrugged (a canine version of a shrug) and went back to inspecting more bins.

I called the number on the card and made an appointment to meet Chris Rungé at our home. The moment she sat down Charley leapt onto her lap and planted herself there as if they were old friends. Chris and I discovered our paths had crossed several times over the years, from horse shows in Pennsylvania to Abadiania, Brazil, where I had gone to interview a famous healer that Chris had also been to see. Seems she knew many of the healers I had written about over the years.

Charley, having spotted something of interest across the room, jumped down from Chris's lap and bounded over to a nest of cables, one of them to my computer.

I stood, ready to grab her.

"Charley, no!" Chris's voice stopped Charley in her tracks and caused her head to snap to attention.

Charley, meet your Alpha match.

Charley was invited to join the assortment of dogs, large and small, old and young, for a few hours a day. Chris would pick up Charley in her SUV, which I came to refer to as the School Bus, loaded with dogs and off they'd go to the dog park or to the walk along the river. I could work until one, have a bite of lunch, run a few errands, then pick up Charley on the way home. Tired and happy, Charley would curl up at my feet while I worked a few more hours. She was fast becoming a writer's dog!

After dinner, playtime. Her favorite was a furry Frisbee with a squeaker inside. She would pick it up, squeak it to get my attention and bring it to me. If I wasn't quick enough to grab it she would toss it up in the air herself, high enough to land on top of a lamp shade.

And best of all, cuddle time. If you've ever been on the receiving end of your pet's prolonged loving gaze and felt a lovely warmth wash over you it was not your imagination. According to a recent study reported in the Science American, you were feeling the effects of the hormone oxytocin (not to be confused with the drug OxyContin), released in both you and your pet. A healing hormone for me, because at my next PET scan I was declared officially in remission.

Christmases happened, six of them, Thanksgivings, Easters and Halloweens, a string of birthdays (we are a big family) happened; a book was finished, another was started, I moved to another apartment; Charley, having become a member of the pack, was a regular at Chris's. We settled into our life together, Charley and I, our bond so strong we could read each other's thoughts. I knew when she was hungry and what food she liked best; she knew when I was tired and needed to lie down. She knew when I was going out (I swear she listened in on my phone conversations), and would look at me with an anxious and forlorn expression that had the desired guilt-inducing effect.

But there was one signal I missed. Soon after her sixth birthday, Charley began to develop seizures. The first one happened in the morning at Chris's. In the middle of playing, she suddenly stopped, her whole body began to shake and she cried out, obviously in pain. After a series of blood and urine tests, Dr. Quan suggested we see a neurologist. Diagnosis: cerebella infarct, a sudden inflammation in the back of the brain which in humans would be a classified as a stroke. The cerebellum is the area of the brain responsible for controlling gait and muscle coordination. Cause unknown. Treatment: steroids and Tramadol for pain, and a watchful eye at all times. Prognosis also unknown. Somehow we learned to live with that, but then a year later Charley had a more violent brush with death.

Grabbed off the end of her leash by a coyote while on one of our routine neighborhood walks and nearly killed, the vet said that Charley must have a powerful guardian angel; the punctures on the left and right side of her chest had missed her vital organs by a hair's breath.

After a period of recovery, Charley and I got on with our lives; her job as muse, mine as writer. I was researching and interviewing healers for this book, learning every day about all manner of surprising and in some instances miraculous healings of animals. The world was set right again. Charley's angel was free to go check on her other wards.

Uh-oh, Angel, wait! Not just yet. One day, while out for our afternoon walk, I noticed that Charley was limping. Thinking she might have stopped stepped on something (a carelessly tossed cigarette butt, a shard of glass) I picked her up and examined her paws. Nothing there. As the day wore on and the limp persisted, I thought she might have pulled a muscle.

But the next day, she couldn't use her left hind leg at all. At first, Dr. Quan didn't know what to make of it. An X-ray showed a dark spot on her spine which could be a herniated disc, or even worse, degenerative Myelopathy: Dreaded DVM. Uncommon in her breed, it is nevertheless progressive and incurable—if that is what she had. As I dug deeper into research, I learned that the disease was similar to ALS or Lou Gehrig's disease in people, which is what my husband died of. No! I shook my fist at the heavens, don't you dare!

According to conventional medicine the only option was surgery, which in light of her history of seizures, would be extremely risky and might not even work. One veterinarian I saw said that Charley would never walk again, and hinted that I should prepare myself. I contacted another vet I knew in New York who after looking at the X-ray and reading the report, agreed. Those voices were having an effect on me.

Late one night after several nights in a row of not sleeping, her condition worsening, I looked deeply into Charley's eyes and asked, "Do you have to leave?" Not getting an answer, I fell asleep with tears in my eyes.

The next morning, Charley stood tall and for the first time in weeks put weight on her left leg. And later that day as I sat working at the computer, her furry Frisbee came flying at me landing squarely on my lap. Karen Becker's shaman's words rang in my ears: "All you need to do," Barbara Harvey had said, "is get out of the way and facilitate their healing response without putting anything toxic into them and they will be fine." I took another look at her diet and decided to give her freshly cooked well-balanced meals, organic treats, a probiotic supplement.

Time to turn to the healers. As true healers will do, they jumped right in, some with offers of treatment, some with suggestions, all of them with absolute assurances that Charley could and would recover. And Charley's angel was right there, this time with a whole army of angels.

I had heard about a chiropractor (see chapter on Eileen Haworth) an hour away; an acupuncturist who makes house calls (see Tony George chapter); Leslie Gallagher (also in this book); energy healer and kinesiologist Jeanette Morris; Bryan Boughman, a people chiropractor who since animals were not permitted in his office met us in the parking lot to give Charley a treatment in the car; Sandie Capelli, a sacro-cranial therapist whom I had written about in a previous book came by and gave Charley a treatment. Carol Komitor in Colorado performed two distance healings, following up with phone calls to check on both me and Charley.

Meantime, Chris, a part-time angel, sent out a clarion call—every healer, for people or animals in her phone book (why not? She said, a healer's a healer): Mary Debono (in the chapter Me and My Best Friend) made several trips to L.A. from San Diego to give both Charley and me treatments; Dr. Gabi Gross, a holistic vet from San Diego who uses hair analysis to make a diagnosis; Claudia Logan, an RN who practices several healing modalities, another acupuncturist, Dr. Arlene Gulio, who works out of the vet's office; Marek Zgirski—a healer visiting the US from Poland; another visiting from San Francisco... No one was safe from Chris's pleas for help.

It is now six months later, and Charley is ninety-percent recovered. If asked which of these healings and treatments worked, I wouldn't be able to say; which would I give up? Not one of them. The same fierce determination I saw in her that drew me to her nine-and-a-half years ago, that same single-mindedness to live life, was I believe what got her through each time illness or injury struck. I learn from her every day.

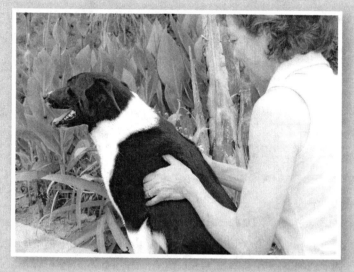

Mary helps Maggie use her back in a healthier way.

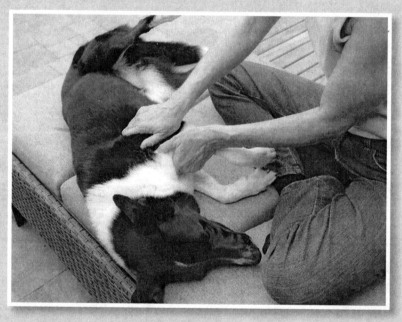

Mary helps Maggie, a canine flyball athlete, release the tension in her shoulders.

PHOTOS: Kathy Upton.

MARY DEBONO

Me and My Best Friend

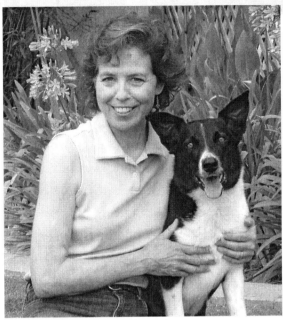

Mary Debono and Maggie.

A little more than a year ago, Charley, my (female) Brussels griffon, was savagely attacked by a coyote. It happened at 7:15 during our morning walk just around the corner from the building where I live. Because I was able to rescue Charley from the coyote's jaws— she needed three surgeries (the gashes missed her vital organs by a millimeter)—miraculously, she survived. Yet, more than a year later, Charley was still showing certain signs of trauma. After it happened, she refused to step off the elevator into the lobby. I had to pick her up and carry her. Once outside on the sidewalk, she was fine, and walking back into the lobby to the elevator was not a problem. Charley's little PTSD, I called it.

I had been hearing about a woman in San Diego County, Mary Debono, whose life and work are devoted to the health and wellbeing of both people and their pets. She is the author of the book, *Grow Young with Your Dog,* which caught my attention.

She writes about how memories of a traumatic injury can become so deeply ingrained that they become habit—in animals as well as in people—and how she works to release those traumas. I wondered if that might apply to Charley. Had Mary Debono found a way to break those habits?

I contacted her and we set up a series of interviews. As it happened, she was due to come to Los Angeles the following week to work on a horse stabled not far from where I live. She offered to come by and demonstrate a few of her exercises.

On a warm bright Saturday morning in early October, Mary arrived at our door carrying her fold-up treatment table. Charley greeted her, tail wagging so hard it was but a blur, and spinning round and round in her happy dance. (Being a writer's dog can get boring.) When we sat, Charley jumped onto her lap and settled there while we talked. Mary gently stroked Charley, introducing her hands to her body.

"To me, the word 'healer,'" she began, "implies that someone outside of ourselves has the power to heal us. I don't feel that way. I feel that I have some knowledge to impart and certain ways of using my hands that with small, gentle movements encourage the muscles to move in new ways. I provide the environment for change, but it's the nervous system itself that makes the changes. My job is to remind the nervous system—human or animal—of what is possible. The healer is within us."

Charley melted beneath her touch, her breathing relaxed and rhythmic as Mary explored the muscles in her neck and along her spine. "This is where she's storing tension," she said, and began to gently move first one and then the other hind leg.

As she continued to work on Charley, I learned her story.

Mary was born in the Bronx, New York. When she was very young, her family, animal lovers all, moved to Long Island where they could have horse property and space for their Norwegian Elkhound. Mary spent a lot of time with her dad, training the dog and going to dog shows, all the while learning to understand more about canine movement and behavior. At seventeen, Mary was given her first horse and was able to expand her burgeoning knowledge.

From the time Mary learned to read, she devoured books about horses and dogs, particularly about the biomechanics of their movements. "At the library, I'd take down all the dog and horse books, as well as human physical therapy books, and spread them out on a big table. I was looking to see how the biomechanics of humans might be applied to animals." These questions led to Mary's exploration of various methods of bodywork with animals: equine massage, acupressure, energy healing, and ultimately, how these methods might relate to humans.

In school, Mary was an honor student. She made honors classes, the Honor Society, and received the school's science award. She certainly could have gone on to college, but her father, who had emigrated from Malta, encouraged her to pursue a business career instead. So, she commuted to a business school in Manhattan, where she became an IT computer programmer. For the next ten years, Mary worked at Wall Street firms, insurance companies, banks, and finally at Credit Suisse in Princeton, New Jersey, amid the rolling hills of beautiful horse country. "But," she recounts, "I had a tremendous amount of responsibility. I had a pager that had to be on 24/7. I would get calls at two in the morning, all day Saturday, and all day Sunday. Or I'd get paged when I was out on my horse, and then have to turn around and run to the office to fix a problem, put out another fire."

All during that time, Mary was plagued by pain, at times severe, in her right hip. It had begun when she was eighteen, puzzling her doctors who, despite various diagnostics, could not explain her symptoms. She was told that by the age of thirty-five, she would probably need a prosthetic hip. Pain became her constant companion, whether working, riding, or sleeping.

To make matters worse, in her later years, Mary developed carpal tunnel syndrome in both hands. The prognosis was grim. A surgeon told her that because the nerves in her arms were so damaged, she would need a series of surgeries followed by steroid injections in her cervical spine. And even then, the most she could hope for was seventy-five percent of her function. Refusing both options, Mary resigned herself to a life of pain. She decided, however, that it would not stop her from pursuing her passion for the study of biomechanics in animals.

One day, as if in answer to unspoken prayers, Mary happened upon an item in a newsletter about a form of therapeutic movement that trains the nervous system to find new pathways around areas of damage, the Feldenkrais Method. Mary read on. Named for its originator, Russian-born physicist Moshe Feldenkrais, the article described its success in rehabilitating stroke victims and those with other neurological injuries. Curious, she called the practitioner mentioned in the article, Lawrence Phillips, to ask for more information. "You have to experience it to really understand it," he explained. She made an appointment for the next day.

"I remember lying on that table, Lawrence moving the muscles on either side of my spine, ribs, and hips very gently, and I could

Mary Debono

actually *feel* changes happening in my body. It was different from anything I had ever experienced.

"I saw him three times a week in the beginning, then as my hip pain gradually subsided, I saw him less and less until eventually the pain disappeared entirely. Lawrence explained that the way I was standing, I was putting so much of my weight on my right hip that my right ribs and hip—the hipbone—were collapsed together, shortening one side of the trunk. That puts strain on that whole area. There are nerves that run out from there, and one can do real damage and develop painful conditions just from those habits.

"People sit crooked, too," Mary explained. "What Lawrence Phillips did for me was enable me to feel—to *recognize*—that it was possible to feel differently than I had been feeling for the past twenty years. And it made me wonder if this technique might work on animals as well.

"Physical therapy for animals was uncommon back then in the late '80s and early '90s, but I had been doing hands-on bodywork with my own and with friends' horses—not professionally, of course—and I had developed my own method of movement education with my hands, some of which came to me intuitively. I kept reading and learning about various methods of bodywork, equine massage, acupressure, and energy work.

"During one of my sessions with Lawrence, I had a sudden overwhelming moment of clarity: I was going to change my life. I was going to learn this work and bring it to the animals.

"As I think back on it, that was a courageous move because I would be giving up a secure financial position and I had a horse that was my dependent. Fortunately, I had saved up some money. A four-year Feldenkrais training was about to start in San Diego; I applied for it, was accepted, and decided I would move there.

17

"This turned out to be a very good thing, because I also met my husband Gary in the training. I noticed him right away—a tall, handsome guy, also a practitioner.

"I soon realized everything I was learning in the training could be applied to animals. When I became a certified practitioner, I called my method 'Debono Moves,' because it's all about moving together with your animal. Something I strive for is to create a loving connection between the individual I am working with and myself, a heart-to-heart connection. Sometimes you might experience that on such a deep level that you will actually feel what they're feeling. And you know it feels right. You engage the heart and the brain. There is a synergy between loving energy and the development of neuroplasticity that helps an individual change and improve—any individual with a nervous system, human or animal. Even an iguana.

"Yes, I once did a session with an iguana. I was called to a woman's house—this is when I used to do house calls. She had four rescued iguanas living in a beautiful big room with gigantic tree branches and an enclosed patio so they could go outside. Seems one of the iguanas had some issues the exotic vet couldn't resolve."

"Iguanas have issues?" I asked.

Mary explained that unlike the other denizens of that odd room, this one was temperamental; he would not allow anyone to approach him, let alone stroke him. In response to my bemused expression, she added that she works on all species, "anything with a nervous system. It's all the same principle."

❧

Mary had also worked with dogs in wheelchairs, a subject dear to me—I had recently written a book, *Miracle Dogs: Adventures on Wheels,* about handicapped dogs. She told me

MARY DEBONO

about one in particular, a male German shepherd suspected of having DM—degenerative myelopathy, a tragic disease common to the breed—who had very little use of his hind legs. "We used the wheels to support his body, then we retrained his brain to use his legs to walk again. We did that by placing his hind paws on top of our feet, and that person would lead him, the way you might teach a child how to dance. I would also use my hands to gently support different parts of his back and his hindquarters to give him reminders that he could use those muscles. These 'neuro-wake-ups' were amazing, because that dog walked on his own again.

"There was another dog, an eight-year-old female Lab mix, that had a severe back injury and had lost all sensation in her hind end. We got her the wheels, which enabled her to stand. Mentally that was good for her, because up until then she had to be carried everywhere. With the help of the wheels, the dog's strength could build gradually, and I was able to adjust accordingly the support needed from the wheels. Gradually, the wheels became almost just a reminder until the dog was able to walk without them."

❧

"My focus is on teaching people how to work on their own with their pets. I find it deepens the bond between human and animal. That's my goal. When I travel, people can either bring their own pets or we can provide animals for them to practice with. Privately, I do work with humans. Three days a week, in Encinitas, I do Feldenkrais sessions, sometimes on Skype.

"I want people to know that there are options to how they're feeling, to know that it's not only possible to feel better physically, but better emotionally and mentally as well, to have a different outlook.

"If you have a dog that isn't using his or her hind legs, for example, you obviously have to think about what's going on. Yes, there's injury. But how much of that is due to habit? Can we create new neuro-connections? How can we do that? We have to be really creative, because we don't want to overwhelm the system. It has to feel safe and pleasurable for the animal. That's the key.

"That's true with people too, because if we tell them, *No, no! Feel the burn, feel the burn,* the nervous system shouts *danger!* And the person goes into protective mode. But if we can keep the process feeling good, eventually the brain will say, 'You know what? This is actually a more efficient and healthier way of sitting/standing/walking/*being.*'"

❧

It was my turn. My issue was my back. Over the years, I had gotten into the habit of writing with my feet up, on the couch, my back propped up against cushions, knees up, notebook or laptop computer on my lap. A chiropractor's dream—or nightmare, depending.

I explained to Mary that I had tried many times, but try as I might, I could not write a single page with my feet on the floor. I got into my pretzel position to demonstrate.

Checking my posture on the couch, she said, "The first thing I would want to do is change the incline." She rearranged the two large, soft cushions behind my back, placing them at a sharper ninety-degree angle, thereby supporting my neck. And by placing a smaller cushion under my knees, the angle of the hips improved. After a few minutes, I told her I could definitely live with those small adjustments.

Next, Mary asked me to lie down on her table. As she had done with Charley, she first explored the muscles and tendons along my spine, then began to test the range of movement of my hips and knees. Her motions were so small and gentle that it was no wonder Charley melted under her touch.

After about 45 minutes, Mary asked me to sit up. I immediately noticed that I was sitting straighter and that my back and chest felt freer and more open.

She also wanted to observe how I walked around the room, asking me to stop at intervals and turn to look over each shoulder. She noticed that it was a little easier for me to turn my head to the left. And that my left leg seemed to stop my movement, which caused my ribcage and spine to stiffen in response.

Mary wondered aloud if the difficulty with my back stemmed more from how I used my legs and pelvis. She explained that the legs and pelvis provide a base of support for the back and ribcage. If their movement is constrained, the trunk muscles often tighten defensively. Standing, she made some additional slight adjustments, then asked me to walk again. Turning to the left was now easier, as my left leg was no longer interfering with the movement of my chest and shoulders. My walking had changed too; it was easier, more stable. Something important had indeed occurred.

❧

Having built a better pretzel, I could now turn my attention back to Charley. I would give Mary's strategy—to provide an opportunity for the pattern to change—a try. Charley was so relaxed after her session with Mary that when it was time for her afternoon walk, instead of picking her up and carrying her across the lobby, I first distracted her with half a treat. Then, just before the elevator doors slid open, I held the other half in front of her nose to lure her out. (I had tried this early on when her PTSD first set in, but to no avail; she would splay herself on the tile floor as if she were glued to it.)

This time Charley took three or four steps out of the elevator before she remembered and slammed to a stop. Quickly, I gave her a piece of the treat and held the rest within sniffing distance as I inched away. Big decision. She half-sat and half-crawled, commando-style, as I inched the treat away. A few more steps, then plunk! Belly on the floor. But as Mary said, "Little moves, big ideas."

We will continue our exercises, my best friend and I, so stay tuned...

❧ ❧ ❧

KATHLEEN PRASAAD

The Light at BrightHaven

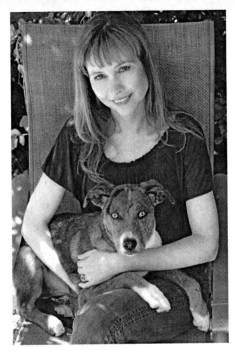

Kathleen Prasaad and Mystic. PHOTO: Lexie Cataldo.

Fifty miles north of San Francisco outside the city of Santa Rosa is an animal sanctuary and hospice, BrightHaven. Founded in the early 1990s by animal rights activists Richard and Gail Pope, whose mission was to save shelter animals most at risk for euthanasia due to age or illness, BrightHaven has also become an extraordinary healing center. Set on ten acres, it functions as a rescue and adoption shelter for abandoned pets and a halfway house for animals as they await adoption. Currently it is home to more than fifty chronically ill and disabled senior animals—dogs, cats, horses, chickens, ducks, a goose, two cows, and a pig. Over the past twenty-five years, the compassionate hospice program has assisted in more than six hundred natural deaths.

In 2005, Kathleen Prasad, author, teacher, and Reiki practitioner, offered to bring the healing technique, Reiki, to BrightHaven, and to teach staff members and volunteers. The Popes accepted, and asked Kathleen to head up the program. To this day, Kathleen remains a part of the family.

Soon after Kathleen arrived, a feral orange tabby cat began to appear at the fence, apparently to visit with Tim, a paraplegic cat who lived there. The two would stand nose to nose, whisker to whisker, apparently communicating through the fence. Staff members, taking notice of the burgeoning friendship, tried to lure the tabby they named Johnny inside, but Johnny would always dart off into the bushes the moment anyone tried to get close to him. Until one crisp autumn day when Johnny decided on his own to slip through the gate to be with Tim. From that day on, the two cats were inseparable, Tim scooting along the ground in his wheelchair, Johnny trotting along beside him.

Staff veterinarians examined Johnny and found a myriad of ailments: renal problems, heart issues, severe dental disease, low potassium, and hyperesthesia. They treated him as best they could; still, they did not expect him to live more than a few months.

At first, the rest of the cat population was not so sure about the newcomer, but before long they began to sense something special about Johnny, and soon he assumed the mantle of top cat. At BrightHaven, a hospice for animals that are in the final chapters of their lives, Johnny would seek out those most in need and sit vigil with each one until the very end.

His attentions didn't stop with animals. At student meetings, he would go around the circle and greet each person. Then, choosing a lap, he'd jump up and gaze into a student's eyes before curling up and falling asleep, purring. For many, it was the first experience of connecting heart-to-heart with an animal.

For others, Johnny's presence ignited a particular healing experience. One student, who had never cried after the recent loss of a parent, gave in to a stream of tears and released weeks of pent-up grieving.

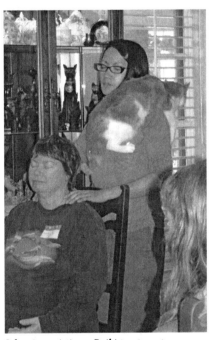

Most of the animals that turn up at BrightHaven have either been slated for euthanasia at the shelters where they were kept, or dropped off by their owners because of a serious terminal illness. Kathleen Prasad says, "But they come to BrightHaven

Johnnie, assisting a Reiki treatment.

and guess what? They live. We see that so often. BrightHaven has a very important recipe: love, natural diet, Reiki, homeopathy, and more love."

She goes on to describe a cat named Frasier, who lived to be over thirty. "He had had cancer for many years, and even lost his eye and part of his face to the disease. But he was the most beautiful, strong spirit that you could ever meet. Frasier loved Reiki. Whenever I came into the room he would run to me and jump on my legs wanting to be picked up. When we were doing the photo shoot for my first book, *Animal Reiki,* and we were photographing all the animals, Frasier wanted to be in every single one. 'OK, Frasier,' I'd tell him. 'You were in the last five pictures. Now I'm going to go sit with the dogs.' Nope, there was Frasier. We'd go out to photograph the horses, and Frasier was right there following after us. He lived for many, many years with cancer, and I do mean, living."

❧

Kathleen Prasad had never been particularly interested in holistic healing; before finding Reiki, her focus was on academics. Born in Berkeley, California, she did her undergraduate studies at Berkeley, majoring in American history, social studies, race relations, and ethnic studies. At graduate school in Sacramento she earned her teaching credentials in English and social studies, and taught language arts and social studies at a middle school. She also ran the drama department.

Her overriding mission was to reach inner-city youths who were at risk and falling through the cracks. At first, the students were tuned out and totally disengaged. Then one day, Kathleen decided to bring photographs of her dogs and cats to class and talk about all the many lonely and forgotten pets in animal shelters. "Suddenly, kids started coming up to my desk to ask me questions and to share something about their own life. At last we had a connection.

"I ended up writing a whole curriculum on kindness to animals, which I incorporated into the program, and asked the class to keep diaries of their activities. As a final project, students were to go into the community and volunteer at shelters. Kids who used to cut school and never finish an assignment were going out on weekends cleaning cages and making videos of what they had done."

Kathleen discovered then the magical effect animals could have on the most tuned-out and disaffected kids. Animals could reach the most unreachable.

"It was right about then that Reiki came into my life. At first, I assumed it was a treatment for an illness. My mother-in-law had a severe post-surgery problem that was corrected after just three Reiki sessions and she urged me to try it. I can't remember if I had a specific issue; I only remember that it felt like a massage times a thousand. I was so relaxed! I felt like I was floating on a cloud. And that feeling stayed with me after I left. I had to know more. I had to learn this!

"It took years of experience and hours and hours of classes before I understood that Reiki is not something you do—it is a state of being. I learned its five precepts: *For today only: do not anger, do not worry, be humble, be honest in your work, and be compassionate to yourself and others.* I learned techniques to become more mindful and to bring all my energies to the present moment. Because when we do that, our heart opens and we're able to connect with others at the heart level.

"Something in me was changing. I was so sure I would be a middle school teacher for the rest of my life, but now I started to wonder how it might be to try Reiki on animals. Back in the '90s and early 2000s, Reiki was still new and intended for humans. But I happened to see a show on PBS about the plight of elephants around the world—I think it was called Urban Elephants—that featured an elephant sanctuary in Tennessee. As I watched, it occurred to me that these elephants, given the conditions they survived, might benefit from Reiki.

"I emailed Carol Buckley, cofounder of the elephant sanctuary, and introduced myself: 'I would love to be of service—to come and teach you Reiki so that you can share it with your elephants.

I would like to do this as a donation to your group for all you do for the elephants of the world.'

"Carol responded right away. 'We're not open to the public, and I don't normally do this, but when I got your email, I felt that you must come here. You *need* to come here.'

"I waited until the end of the school year, just before I retired, and asked Elizabeth Fulton, coauthor of my first book, to come with me. During the four or five days of our visit to Tennessee, I gave Carol and a few of her employees a demonstration of Reiki. We were allowed to meet some of the elephants, but not to work directly on them; only people who are going to actually be in their life are allowed to work with them. Elephants are very sensitive creatures and they really bond with people: it's stressful for them to meet somebody and then have that person leave. But we were able to see them in their natural habitat, roaming free in the field. When you see all animals as spiritual beings and you open your heart to them, you understand how desperately needed these animal sanctuaries and their caregivers are.

"After that, I dove into private practice and taught classes —some at Guide Dogs for the Blind, some at the local Berkeley Animal Care Services where I volunteered. I remember a very sick, eighty-pound pit bull I treated. They brought him to me in a small private room where I worked. The poor thing was shaking uncontrollably and so scared he couldn't even walk upright; he was crawling like a lizard with his belly on the ground.

"I never go put my hands on an animal. I always let the animal come to me. So, I sat with my hands in my lap and waited. When finally, he came over to me, he curled himself up into a ball. After a while, I put my hands on him and did the Reiki meditation of love and kindness. He soaked it up. At some point during the treatment he began to shake uncontrollably again. Then he released, took a big sigh and fell asleep. I sat with him for about an hour more. When he woke up, I put him on his leash and he stood like any normal dog. I walked him over to the staff's office, and said, 'He's all done, you can take him back to his kennel.' They couldn't believe he was the same dog. And that was just one treatment.

"Not every animal responds after just one treatment, but he did. There were so many times when dogs that were completely stressed out would totally relax, and when dogs that were almost completely checked out would suddenly get the light back in their eyes. *This is it*, I thought. *This is what we need to heal the world!*"

❧

Years later, after several years of teaching at BrightHaven, Kathleen faced her own health challenge. "After my surgery for breast cancer, when I returned to BrightHaven, it was that wonderful orange tabby Johnny who came running to me. He jumped right up onto my lap and stretched his entire body over my shoulder and across my chest, purring loudly. I closed my eyes and relaxed,

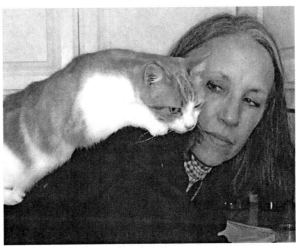

Johnnie, always lending a healing paw. PHOTO: BrightHaven.

29

allowing him to do his healing on me. As Johnny's breathing grew more relaxed and regular, I could feel a lessening of my post-surgical pain. He and I could both let go of our health issues and just be present together in that beautiful, peaceful space.

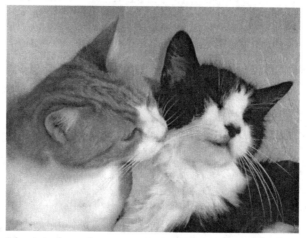

Johnnie is always there to support animals as well as people.
PHOTO: BrightHaven.

"Johnny taught me that true and lasting healing is not about curing this or that problem. We can be truly healed, or made whole, when we let go of the need to cure and instead simply connect to others from the heart with selfless compassion. It's then that we create a space where all healing potential exists, and miracles of healing can occur!

"Johnny passed away after a long journey of healing so many others, even with his own many health issues. He had a peaceful passing surrounded by loved ones, just as he had sat vigil in hospice for others so many times."

❦

These days, Kathleen has a full schedule: she continues to teach classes both at BrightHaven and at partner sanctuaries

KATHLEEN PRASAD

around the world. She facilitates her online education and tele-class program, speaks at international conferences, and runs her nonprofit Shelter Animal Reiki Association. She has little time for her private practice. "The first seven or eight years of my full-time practice I went to people's barns or their homes. But now, because my schedule is so busy, I offer distant treatments.

"In Reiki teachings, there is really no such thing as distance, because distance is just a perception. We're all one, all connected. It's only when we forget this connection that we feel separate. If we're all one, it means that everything is right here already; within the oneness we create the healing space. So, it's not like I am really sending Reiki here or there, or reaching across the world to do a healing; I'm going inward into my heart and remembering that it all resides within me already."

꿱

Each February, Kathleen teaches healing at an exotic animal sanctuary in Florida where tigers, bears, and snakes reside. "Talk about the wisdom of Mother Earth and the ancient wisdom. I mean, those snakes! When you connect with them it's incredible! They're safely in their little cage; I sit outside and practice my Reiki. This past September, I went to Animal Haven in New York City, a shelter in SoHo where we were being filmed for a TV show performing Reiki on the shelter animals.

"For me, it's really about the spirit and compassion, and that underneath our differences of species, we're really the same. True healing is about healing our spirit and remembering that we are all one. Because, in reality, we're all going to die. This body will not last forever. Who we are is eternal. That beautiful bright light that exists within all of us, human and animal, is always there, it's always perfect, and it goes on."

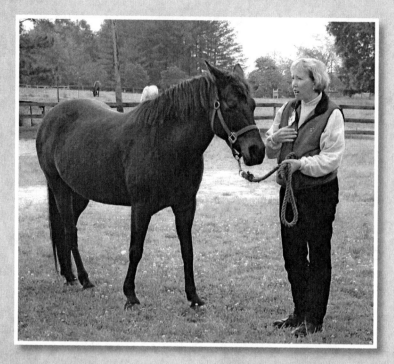

Carol explains how to work with severe conditions such as proud flesh.

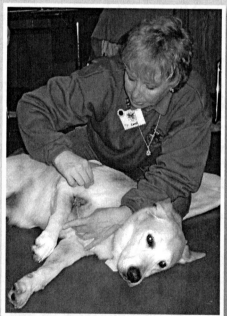

Carol uses Healing Touch for Animals® technique during classroom demonstration.

CAROL KOMITOR

A Voice for all God's Creatures

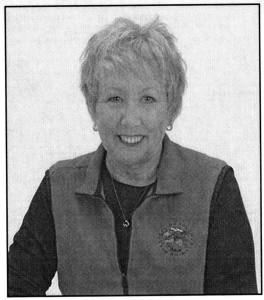

Carol Komitor, founder of Healing Touch for Animals.

C arol Komitor, founder and director of Healing Touch for Animals, believes her purpose in life is to be a voice for the animals. "Because if they become extinct, we will, too. We are only one small part of the whole of life on this planet; animals are its heart and soul, especially domestic animals. Whether a dog, a cat, a guinea pig, or a goldfish in a bowl that lives on the kitchen counter like mine and does a little dance whenever I walk by, they all come from a place of unconditional love.

"Animals have a much larger field of energy than humans—at least ten times larger—therefore they're more receptive, more sensitive to their surroundings than we are. When our pet is sitting next to us, we are inside their field. If we're having a bad day, if we're emotionally upset or physically ill, our animals take that into their field. The problem is, sometimes they hold onto that stress, which can create illness for them. And considering all the turmoil in the world around us from financial to relationships to world communities fighting against each other, we humans are constantly dealing with stress. Stress affects our adrenals, which in turn affects our immune system, making it difficult for both us and our pets to fight off disease."

Having begun her career as a veterinary technician, Carol saw firsthand cases of a person with diabetes whose dog also had diabetes, and someone with cancer whose animal developed cancer. "At the time, I didn't know anything about energy medicine, I just thought it was an interesting coincidence. After more than twenty years of practice, I've learned otherwise. As animal healers, we have to let those animals know it is not their job to take on anything that does not belong to them. We can do that by talking to them—not that they actually understand the words (although some do), but they do read our energy field. Just as they can discern what we're feeling, whether it's joy or love, or sadness or fear.

"We have a contract with our domesticated animals: in return for food and shelter and companionship, they give us their loyalty and unconditional love. Dogs are heart based—when I work with them I can see their energy going directly to the heart of their owners. Cats have a more expanded awareness: a telepathic ability that encompasses our entire environment—our house and our property and wherever it is we happen to be. Our horses are flight animals, they love their people and they embrace them as part of their herd, but people must be the leaders in the horse herd so they don't get trampled.

"Regarding our animals in the zoo, their contract with us is to let people see the beauty of who they are so that we'll campaign to save them."

As seems to be the case with many healers, Carol was no stranger to personal health problems. As a child, she was shy and sickly, having endured a series of surgeries to correct her eyes, which were severely crossed.

In later years, as a busy single mom, her immune system depleted, she developed a sinus infection that she couldn't seem to get rid of... until the day she had a treatment with a therapist who incorporated a certain kind of energy facilitation called "Healing Touch" with the massage, and Carol's life changed. Suddenly she felt a powerful shift, one that led her to an exploration of energy work. "I set out to find a Healing Touch class and met Janet Mentgen, a well-known holistic nurse who invented the Healing Touch system, and I enrolled in her course."

As fellow participants in the program became aware of Carol's thirteen years of experience as a veterinarian technician, they began to turn to her with questions about whether Healing Touch might work on animals. Carol explained that although the chakras are essentially the same in animals as they are in humans, working with animal energy would be different in that their energy fields are much larger than those of humans, making them even more receptive.

During an extended break at an advanced Healing Touch course, she took the other students outside to the field where a horse was kept and pointed to where the specific energy centers were in the horse's body. She explained, "We humans have layered systems that encompass our physical, emotional and mental bodies. In animals, that system is integrated, not layered, like little pixels in a digital picture that encompass the animal's electromagnetic field. They are able to expand that energy field to ten times greater, enabling them to read us a whole lot better than we can read them. That instinctual field gives them the information needed for a fight or flight response."

After she received her certification and completed her hospital-based massage training, Carol's first massage client was a cancer patient. "I saw her through three bouts of different types of cancers, and to this day she is living and doing well. Word got around, and at one point, eighty percent of my clientele, both animals and people, were cancer patients. And even as we provided the best of their care, we were able to learn from them, too. Most were very receptive and open to the work. I've seen everything: from absolute miracles to helping a person peacefully transition in their end-of-life stages."

As interest in animal care among her colleagues continued to grow, Carol decided to develop a course of her own to address the animal aspect of Healing Touch. Carol explains, "Our work creates relaxation. When an animal is relaxed, endorphins in the brain are released and the muscles open, allowing more circulation and blood to flow through the body. That brings in oxygen and nutrients, and distributes the enzymes needed for proper digestion. It also flushes out toxicity and helps to promote healthy cell growth. The major thrust of what our work does is to help support the immune system so that the body can heal itself."

With regards to behavioral issues, and asked how she deals with animal aggression, Carol describes a technique she calls, "bridging." "First, we balance the energy system, then we use a script about their behavior and what changes must be made, letting them know if some behavior they're exhibiting is inappropriate and has to stop. Then we give them a "job." That job might be that they become an elegant leader in the herd, or to respect the people who take care of them. Within the household, their job is to understand that all life must be respected. That includes property, the people, and all other living beings in the household. In return, they receive unconditional love and care, from food and shelter to loving companionship.

"Sometimes an animal needs direction just like a human teenager does, and we need to reroute the path they're headed down. Because inappropriate behavior is not their true expression; it's a cry of 'Hey, pay attention to me,' or 'I'm going to get my own way because I don't know what other way to go.' I don't claim to be an animal communicator, but I do know that in working with the energy system we can communicate and receive droves of information.

"With direction, and with the balance that we create for them, along with their own keen awareness, changes occur quickly and easily. We never use the old 'cowboy' approach, we never use fear techniques. I didn't used to speak out loud to the animal. You don't have to, but I do now so that the animal's owner can more easily help support the changes being made."

Carol describes the class: "Before the work can really begin, the facilitator must be grounded and clear, setting the atmosphere for the highest and best intention. Then, we center ourselves and find the quiet place within. Being centered is to be consistent and mindful. Setting the intention means we must hold the highest purpose for the animal. Then, you develop a plan of treatment using the Healing Touch for Animals (HTA) techniques to determine which will be most helpful for your subject. And finally, you must put yourself in 'allow' mode, letting the energy flow into the body. Energy follows intention, so by allowing the energy to flow, it regulates itself."

During a session, the facilitator can use one of several HTA techniques to specifically address a variety of issues. For example, a bridging technique is often used for animals that are scattered or fragmented due to illness, injury, or personality disorder. This technique balances and clears the energy field and brings wholeness into place.

"Once you are centered, place one hand on the chest at the animal's heart chakra, the other in front of the withers on the throat chakra. As the energy runs through you into the animal, you send your message with words or thoughts to them, pausing with your words between each step as you facilitate the energy flow. Balance the energy system for ten to twenty minutes before you begin the script. Focusing on the balance first creates a better foundation for change."

She illustrates with five points:

1. Communicate the inappropriate behavior: "You are destroying the furniture when I'm gone."
2. Clarify your expectations: "I expect this to stop."
3. Give your pet a job: "Your new job is to keep an eye on the house when I'm gone and to help create peace and harmony in our household. I appreciate your loyal companionship."
4. Provide support: "You are loved and supported in this new job."
5. Tell them they need to "remember." The word remember taps into the energy balance that was created with the bridging technique, but it also connects to the words that were offered. Use the actual word "remember" when they act out.

Beginning twenty years ago with just a couple of classes in Denver, Healing Touch for Animals is now an international, multilevel program that leads to certification. HTA instructors currently offer workshops worldwide. Participants in the weekend workshops learn not only how to forge stronger connections with their animals, but also how to treat behavioral and psychological issues.

Carol's popularity, however, was not without its challenges: conventional veterinary medicine was not always accepting of her methods. And even though she knew she had something important to offer, she found it difficult "not to just melt into the wallpaper." The woman who was determined to help animals find their voice had to find hers as well.

"I see our work as a cooperative measure. Our doctors and nurse practitioners have technology that can diagnose well beyond anything we can. The veterinarians can use their diagnostic tools, perform surgery and prescribe medications. What I am able to do is balance and clear and stabilize the energy system that supports the physical and emotional form. Therefore, working with conventional medicine is a win-win because it creates a viable team for total wholeness."

❧

Two of the animals she's currently working with each have cancer: one, an eight-year-old golden retriever named Tellie who lives with her family outside Vail in Colorado. Tellie was diagnosed with an aggressive osteosarcoma of the jaw, considered terminal. Mikki, a property manager, was desperate. Tellie was hers and her husband's first dog and they were devoted to her. After extensive research online, Mikki came upon Carol Komitor's work. Although the concept of healing was foreign to

Mikki, especially over a distance, she read on. Something about the simplicity of Carol's explanation—that a healer was a conduit for the energy that promotes the body's ability to heal itself—appealed to Mikki. Recently, her close friend's dog with a similar cancer was treated with chemo and had died twelve months later; consequently, Mikki was open to explore alternative treatment.

She contacted Carol and they began a series of six sessions. Carol's treatment included the use of essential oils Copaiba and Frankincense, which Tellie would lick off Mikki's hand. Carol also suggested a brew of turmeric, garlic, and ginger cooked with bone marrow. By the end of three months, Tellie's tumor had shrunk to one-fourth its previous size.

Mikki and Tellie continued to attend Carol's weekend classes, and as of this writing, December 2015, Tellie's condition continues to improve.

Deborah Gotto, a graphic designer based in Denver, tells the story of her horse Strider: "Six years ago, Strider was diagnosed with ring bone, a degenerative arthritis disease in which the joints begin to calcify. Strider was limping badly and was clearly in pain. The vet put him on several kinds of pain medications and told us in two years he would probably have to be put down."

Deborah tried a regimen of glucosamine, chondroitin, MSM, and omega-3 fatty acids to help ease the arthritis, but saw little difference. Then she began to practice HTA techniques on Strider, and as her ability progressed, Deborah began to see changes in its effect on her horse. "In Level 4, I learned about the hara line, an energy pipeline that connects to the universe and the Earth. If that energy isn't flowing correctly, it can cause illness. Strider's was blocked," she says. "Once this energy was cleared, Strider was able to receive the work on a deeper level. Deborah worked on Strider at least three times a week using various techniques, and he began to visibly heal. "Now, his limp is almost gone, and I'm taking him on trail rides."

Deborah speculates that an early trauma was the cause of Strider's blocked energy patterns. "As a baby, he was forcibly weaned," she says. "He tried to jump a fence to get back to his mother and his back legs got hung up in the fence. From the first, I wanted to train him to be a jumper, which puts a lot of stress on the legs and feet, as well as mentally. I think both those two things caused a great deal of trauma." Deborah believes this led to the energy congestion that, combined with a genetic predisposition to ring bone, provoked the disease.

"Blockages make illness manifest earlier," Deborah says, but HTA can counteract these effects by balancing the immune system. "You have to believe in what you're doing, work with it, and be consistent about it. You can't go into working on an animal with your own agenda," she says. "I wanted to heal the ring bone, but a lot of other things happened that I didn't expect. Strider's always been a spook, but that flight response has settled. He trusts me now, and we have a really strong bond. He's more like a dog."

And speaking of dogs, Deborah also uses HTA techniques to treat her nine-year-old black Lab, Indy, who suffers from an infiltrative lipoma, a tumor that penetrates into the muscles and nerves and chokes off blood and oxygen supplies. The lipoma was on Indy's hind leg and had spread throughout his entire upper thigh, creating large protrusions both on top of and underneath the leg. Conventional treatment is most often amputation, which Deborah refused to consider. "Within three days of the HTA therapies, Indy was using that leg again," she says. "The lipoma is now much smaller and seems to be continually shrinking. And most importantly, Indy's back to playing and being a dog again."

Indy had also suffered from another lipoma on his chest where he'd been kicked by a horse. When she began working on Indy's leg, Deborah noticed that the lipoma on his chest had also begun to shrink. "It was about the size of a small grapefruit; now it's reduced to the size of a golf ball. I don't expect it to be gone for months, maybe a year, but it is dissolving."

Deborah now works alongside Carol, helping to organize classes and designing materials. And she continues to work on both Strider and Indy.

Since Carol's children are both grown and have careers of their own, she is free to travel to teach her classes. When she's not traveling, she sees clients in person and does coaching sessions and distance work over the phone. She also distributes essential oils for her preferred brand.

"To be an emotional support for animals through their energetic field is a wonderful job, a privilege for those of us whose lives are dedicated to their health and well-being. I am proud to be among the voices that speak for their continued safety and existence on the planet."

KAREN BECKER

The Shaman's Apprentice

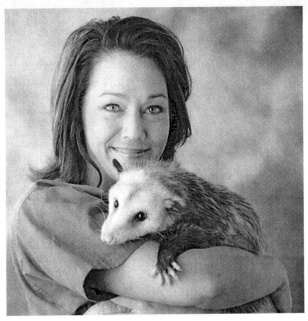

Dr. Becker with educational opossum, Clara.

Karen Becker knew from a very early age that she was put on this earth to care for life in all its many forms. Born with a hearing impairment, one of her earliest memories is going outside in the rain at the age of three to pick up the worms from the sidewalk to rescue them from drowning. She would take care of them, hundreds of them, until the sun came out, and then she would carefully place them back outside in the grass. She believes that being hearing impaired allowed her to absorb the natural world with one less sense that was, for her, one less distraction.

Growing up in Cedar Falls, Iowa, Karen's entire focus was on caring for animals that needed help. Her parents, both teachers, allowed her to bring home any and all wounded or ill creatures— from turtles with broken shells to snakes, bugs, frogs, lizards, and baby bunnies.

"When I looked at a bird with a broken wing, I felt so helpless. I didn't know where to turn to get help—there was no Internet back then. My parents, realizing early on that I had a deep connection with all things wild, facilitated my dream of becoming a wildlife rehabilitator."

By thirteen, determined to find the best training, Karen discovered the Black Hawk Humane Society in Waterloo, Iowa, a facility that took in orphaned and injured wildlife; she called to ask to volunteer. Her boss there, Tom Colvin, took her under his wing and became her mentor, marking the beginning of Karen's honing her skills. At fourteen she became a state-licensed wildlife rehabilitator; by sixteen, she was federally licensed.

"One day I read a journal article about a woman who had the nation's top rehabilitation success rate—ninety percent, which was unheard of. The average national success rate was about thirty-three percent. I found her number and called her, explaining who I was and what I was doing. 'My success rate is thirty percent,' I said, 'but I heard about *your* success rate and I'd like to know more.'

"Barbara Harvey was frank with me. 'The reason you're having such a terrible success rate is that you're poisoning your animals; they were thriving and vital until they became injured. All you need to do is get out of the way and facilitate their healing response without putting anything toxic into them and they will be fine,' she said. And then the phone went dead! Thinking we had been disconnected, I called her back. 'Barbara, I think we got disconnected.'

"'No, I hung up.'

"'But why?' Keep in mind that I had just turned fourteen. Now, at forty-five, if someone hung up on me I would just think maybe they'll call back in a year or two or ten, and I would let it go. But at fourteen, I didn't know to let it go. 'Barbara, I'm really hurt that you would hang up on me. I'm calling because I want to have a high success rate like yours. I'd like to come and visit.'"

Somehow Karen was able to talk her parents into driving her to Horicon, a little town in Wisconsin two hundred and fifty miles away. "To this day I razz my mother, 'I cannot believe you drove a fourteen-year-old child to a stranger's home in another state and just dropped her off.' In this day and age, you'd never do that.

"Barbara was waiting for us in the middle of the driveway as we pulled into her wooded sanctuary. A thin, tiny woman with long, straight, raven-black hair and impeccable posture, she had an aura of calm confidence about her I had not seen in any other person."

It was spring. Barbara, who was half Native American—Mohawk on her mother's side—had a teepee in her front yard where she slept in warm weather. She used her log cabin only in winter. That night, she announced to Karen that they would be sleeping in the teepee.

As Karen vividly recalls, "Barbara did not engage in small talk or chitchat. Her words were chosen carefully and she often spoke in metaphors. My never-ending questions were often answered with Native-American poetry. By not giving me direct answers and instead giving me so much food for thought, she accomplished two goals: she shut me up (because my head was so full) and she provided lasting, timeless answers I would draw upon decades later.

"My parents had just pulled out of the driveway when Barbara turned to me and said, 'Let's go to the Mouse House.'"

The Mouse House was a heated and cooled outdoor rodent-breeding facility. On the inside of all the cages were cutouts from *National Geographic*. Karen asked about them.

"'Mice and rats are incredibly smart; while they are here on earth they need a lot of environmental enrichment, so I provide them things to do during the day and beautiful things to look at (hence the pictures inside their cages). But they also know their role here. They know why I breed them, and since they are in the food supply, their energies will be transferred up the food chain. During their life on earth, I want them to be happy, healthy animals—happy, healthy energy, which translates into happy, healthy food. We don't want our mice and rats to be bored or stressed out or have a miserable life, because that would transfer up the food chain.

"'So, lesson number one: Your animals are the food that they eat. If they eat dead, inorganic, and processed food or frozen dead food, that will hinder their healing response. Don't ever buy frozen mice for injured raptors. That's junk food. Live food is what nature intended for them to eat, especially when they're sick, diseased, or injured. Vibrant bodies are the result of vibrant food.'

"Barbara opened up a cage of rats and held her hand out. 'Okay,' she announced, 'I'm going to accept volunteers.'

"The first rat climbed into her hand. In her other hand, she held a five-gallon bucket into which she put the rat. As she thanked volunteer number one, volunteer number two came up to her. She did not pick it up by the tail, which is what I had always seen done, because when you pick up animals that are going to be food, you want to grab them quickly, so as not to get bitten.

"The next rat stepped forward and crawled onto her hand. Gently, she placed that one into the bucket as well. Now she needed some mice, so she closed that bin and opened the next. 'Okay,' she called out, 'today's the big day! Who wants to transfer energy today?' She got three eager volunteers.

"After that, we went outside and stood behind two giant pine trees. She called out something in her native tongue and waited; we just stood there, waiting in silence. It felt like we stood there forever.

"Finally, I looked at her and asked, 'Barbara, what are we doing?'

"She shushed me. 'Be quiet.'

"'Barbara'—I was an impatient fourteen-year-old. 'We're just standing here. What are we doing?'

"'We're calling in our guests.'

"'How? You're not saying anything.'

"'Ach! You have so much to learn. Be quiet!'

"So, I just stood there for what felt like a flipping eternity.

"Finally, she said, 'Okay, are you ready?'

"I had no idea for what. 'Yes.'

"Barbara reached into the pail, grabbed a mouse, and chucked it into the air. Out of the blue a snowy owl swooped down and grabbed the mouse midair.

"All five of our volunteers had a raptor waiting, and all those raptors got lunch that day. Those mice were fired up to volunteer, to go back to pure positive energy. It was the strongest display of energy that I have ever seen in my life."

Karen pauses in telling this story, her voice filled with emotion. "I am an avian orthopedic surgeon and I do a lot of bone repair on birds. I need you to know that even with twenty years as an avian veterinarian under my belt, this woman, this healer,

Barbara Harvey, without surgery, without a degree, was able to fix things that to this day make me shudder, things that I have apprehensions about even trying to fix.

"Barbara showed me early on that working with an animal's body often means unlocking the body's healing potential and getting out of the way; the actual magic of healing is contained within the body itself. It also means communicating your wants and your desires to that animal very, very clearly.

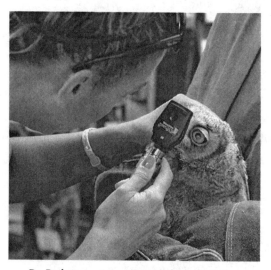

Dr. Becker examining an injured Screech owl.

"I came home from that experience a very different girl. I saw wild animals cooperate and interact with a human as a result of an energetic relationship that I did not know was possible. What I learned from this woman in one week was life-altering. I saw her move energy in a way that connected so clearly with wild animals. She *commanded* energy. *Directed* energy. There were owls, hawks, and falcons that she had rehabilitated years ago that were still living on her property and were free to come and go. They were not imprinted, they just had a very deep relationship with her and chose to stay.

❧

"Barbara Harvey provided a lifetime of learning opportunities in that one week of living with her. She sent me home with a tackle box full of homeopathic remedies. I had never heard of the word 'homeopathy' before; I didn't know what it was. She told me that homeopathic remedies are very much diluted, all-natural substances made from plants, minerals, and other organic and inorganic materials that do not harm any of the wildlife, and have the potential to help them heal faster. She had written a little cookbook for me which, now as a licensed veterinary homeopath, I realize that you are not supposed to do. But she knew I needed the recipes. For instance, she wrote that for a poked-out eye, give Ledum, which is a homeopathic remedy for eye trauma. 'If an animal comes in with a broken wing, give Arnica, followed by Symphytum. If an animal is in shock, give Aconite.'"

That following summer, Karen's success rate went from thirty-eight percent to fifty percent; the next year to sixty-five percent; the year after that to eighty-five percent. "I thought it would take forever, but the speed of my success was the direct result of the profound wisdom that Barbara had shared with me.

"The first time I had ever heard any type of negative comment about homeopathy was when I was eighteen and was asked to give a lecture at the National Wildlife Rehabilitators Association. I was explaining the different homeopathic remedies I was using when someone said, 'You understand that that's voodoo, right?'

"'What?'

"'You understand there's no real medicine in homeopathic remedies. It's diluted out so many times that there's nothing left. You are practicing voodoo.'

"I recognized then that homeopathy was just the first of many modalities that I had in my tool bag that would not be widely accepted."

The University of Wisconsin-Stevens Point has an entire College of Natural Resources dedicated to soil, water, forestry, and wildlife. Karen's goal was to be a wildlife biologist, but she also wanted to continue honing her rehab skills. In her freshman year, frustrated that she didn't have a medical background, she decided to shift her focus. "My parents were not wealthy, so I could not afford to go to vet school out of state. I applied to Iowa State and was accepted, thank God. I headed back to Ames, Iowa, to complete my veterinary degree training.

"Two nights before I started vet school, Barbara Harvey called me. 'Karen, I'm going to tell you this, and I'm only going to tell you this once. They are going to try and pollute your brain. And I want you to know that if you are like the other young veterinarians that I have mentored, you'll come out not only questioning homeopathy, you'll come out saying "Barbara, I can't believe that you still believe in all this." You know who you are in your soul, and I know that you may come out having more questions. But I also know you are never going to forget what you saw.'

"'Barbara, I will never forget what I saw.'

"She checked in with me regularly, all through my four years of vet school. That's when the challenges became very real. In pharmacology class, we were taught about morphine and all the morphine derivatives. It seemed logical to me to raise my hand and ask, 'What about when pain meds don't work and there are side effects? What do you do when you have a patient that desperately needs pain meds but can't tolerate the drugs?'

"By the time I graduated I had raised quite a ruckus! I am not by nature a person who likes to stir the pot, but sitting for four years in vet school I sometimes had some burning questions. I was sent down to the dean's office to discuss my behavior on many occasions.

"During my orthopedics lab, they wanted me to fracture the leg of a healthy beagle and then pin it back together. And I said I was sorry, but I was not going to fracture a healthy bone. Off I went to the dean's office. Then, in my senior year, when I wanted to take veterinary acupuncture training as my elective study, the dean denied my request, so I went to the board with my request.

"When I had my exit interview—that's when the dean calls in every graduating veterinarian to reflect on their time at the school—the dean said, 'Karen, I don't want to hear anything out of you. But I will tell you this one thing: I have never been so glad to see a student go. You are not welcome back as long as I'm dean. You have too many questions that veer off into non-science. This is a technical institute. We're graduating doctors, not shamans!'

"I've since been back to Iowa State to give lectures. And I have to admit that I remember, with a silly grin on my face, how the dean (who is no longer there) banned me. Yet here I am, teaching brilliant young students how to open their minds. Karma is awesome, eh?"

However, those challenges continued to follow her after veterinary school. While readily acknowledging that conventional medicine is "flipping awesome—if you get hit by a bus," Karen is quick to point out its limitations. "When it comes to chronic and lifestyle diseases, or emotional diseases that lead to a physical disease, and we look at the underlying causes of these ills, we can see that medicine in the United States has failed. I think we are far behind other countries—in both human and veterinary medicine."

She reminds us that veterinarians have an extra challenge because their patients can't talk. "We have to rely on body language and reading our patients, not just their facial expressions but also things like the position of their ears and eyes, as well as their respiration rate. You can see when a patient starts breathing shallowly. You can see by their twitchiness that they're nervous. Different animals have different sets of characteristic behaviors that will tell you how they're doing emotionally. In snakes, the tongue flicks communicate information to us; turtles and birds express feelings through their eyes. How do we assess pain in those animals? How do we assess previous emotional trauma that is causing a non-healing wound? How are we assessing those parameters? We're not."

What needs changing, Karen believes, is the whole approach to education. "We don't have classes on stewardship or fostering empathy. We don't have classes that teach animal body language, the natural history, behaviors, and diets of the animals we keep as pets, or about the interconnectedness of life. I don't believe we are preparing future generations to be active, integrative components in an ecosystem that desperately needs their committed stewardship. The earth is wearing out right now, partially from abuse, partially from neglect. And the levels of toxins are becoming dangerously high.

"At the same time, our soils have been degraded to the point that they are no longer sustainable. We have chunks of earth that are literally dead, no longer viable for growing or sustaining any type of life, plant or animal. Still, I think that as long as our hearts continue to beat on this planet, we can grow and evolve and change.

"I would say that the most important aspect of my being a healer is not necessarily related to my degree. While it affords me the opportunity to have a broader reach, my goals as a veterinarian—a holistic veterinarian—remain identical to my goals as a healer of wildlife. Many veterinarians are conventionally trained, but without enough tools in their toolbox. By the first or second year of practice, most of us realize that even though we are diagnosing and treating animals exactly as we were taught, no one told us what to do when animals don't respond as described in the textbooks. You can do everything exactly right. You can suture the wound, you can prescribe the right medication for the right period of time at the right concentration, and you still have patients that don't heal. They didn't teach us in vet school what Plans B, C, D, and E might be. As a holistic practitioner, I had to come up with those next steps myself.

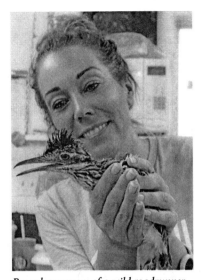

Pre-release exam of a wild roadrunner.

"One of my goals is to provide educational opportunities for practitioners and for pet parents who might have had a dog or cat die prematurely of a preventable disease. My outreach is to everyone who wants to grow and evolve and become better caretakers of our animals.

"I am by nature a terrier of a person: type A, goal-oriented, and definitely a go-getter. Twenty years ago, whether people knew they needed the information or not, I was hell-bent on giving it to them. I've evolved enough now to realize that some may not be ready for this information right now, and that's okay. But for those who have come to a receptive point in their own personal evolution, my goal is to connect them with people who will facilitate their learning."

❧

Karen divides her time between her homes in Chicago and Arizona. In 1999, she opened her own animal hospital in the Chicago area, Natural Pet; in 2002, she founded Covenant Wildlife Rehabilitation, a not-for-profit, organization dedicated to caring for injured wild animals. The organization provides care to over 200 wild animals each year, free of charge. Karen feels strongly that wild animals must be valued and cared for as vital members of our ecosystem, from sparrows to eagles, bunnies to beavers.

Also in 2002, she founded Feathers Bird Clinic, an exotic animal practice; in 2011, she started Therapaw Canine Rehabilitation and Pain Management Center.

"I sold Natural Pet in 2013 because I was having a hard time

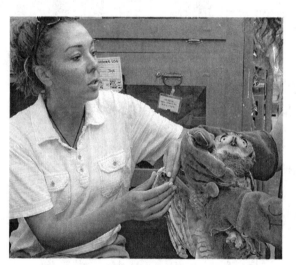

Physical therapy on a Great Horned owl.

finding enough hours in a day. I was in the exam room eight to ten hours a day, leaving little time for anything else. Now I work there part-time, which gives me time to write and lecture." Karen has written three pet cookbooks, among them the award-winning *Whole Dog Journal,* published in 2009. She also hosts the largest online pet wellness website in the world, www.healthypets.mercola.com, where millions of pet lovers receive her free daily pet health newsletter.

"When I'm not in Arizona, my family takes care of all the critters. When I'm in Chicago, my niece Blair and her two dogs, Buster and Gibbs, live in the house with me. She also adopted a kitty I found in a ditch while driving to work 10 years ago. He had been hit by a car and had a degloving wound that removed all the skin off his left rear limb. He clearly had been there many days as the leg was gangrenous and he was very thin and dehydrated. The 'standard of care' was to amputate these 'unsalvageable' limbs, but I had just heard of doctors using manuka honey (honey made from the manuka or tea tree that has significant antibacterial properties) in third world countries to successfully treat gangrene. I decided to try it on the cat. Once a day I slathered his leg with the honey and applied a light dressing. I started him on aggressive fluid therapy and pain medication. Slowly, he grew new skin and finally hair. I was quite convinced his nails would not regrow because the bones had been exposed for so long that they were black. But he even regrew some toenails! It took him three months to recover, and by that time we had all fallen in love with him. We named him Manuka, and Blair adopted him.

"Then there's Ada and Violet, both pit bulls, twelve and thirteen, and a very silly miniature dachshund. My husband and I stumbled across a homeless dachshund three years ago and we named him Lennie. Cordelia, my educational opossum, just died of old age ten days ago. I have a fondness for misunderstood animals—I call them the 'loathsome species' that humanity hates. Opossums are among the most misunderstood creatures on the planet. I took my toad back to Chicago because it's a little too hot for him in Arizona. And then there are the two great kitties, Enzo and Crosno, that came through the rescue program at Natural Pet.

"My goal is for all animals to be happy, happy, happy, happy— and then to easily transition without deterioration or degeneration. I know that this is possible. That's exactly how both Toady (not a very original name for a toad) and Cordelia died this past year. Both had a beautiful life, and then they had an amazing death. I am thankful for both of those things. I feel that I have done my job as caretaker of the animals that I have been entrusted to.

"My work has changed me in lots of ways. I am by nature not a patient girl; I have had to learn the art of patience. Conventional colleagues refer their patients to integrative veterinarians when they literally have nothing left to offer, and they know that the animal is dying. When I get those cases, I see it as an opportunity. The referring vets may perhaps learn and grow, and at least be open-minded to what I am going to suggest. I know I love learning from healers in a variety of different realms.

"I think sometimes the Universe provides these challenging opportunities for our own personal evolution. I can hear somewhat adequately now because of a number of extensive surgeries when I was younger, and I know that this adversity has made me a better, more astute doctor. I am very sensitive to energy; I can read body language from a mile away.

"I'm still in the exam room and I'm doing consulting work for organic pet food manufacturers. I'm still rehabbing. I have this beautiful blend right now of writing and lecturing, and a little bit of everything else to accomplish my goal of changing the world."

In September of 2016, two weeks before her seventy-seventh birthday, Karen's beloved mentor and shaman, Barbara Harvey, passed away. At her side was her best friend and animal spirit guide, Sasha, her thirty-three-year-old permanently injured red-tailed hawk (the oldest living documented red-tail), and Barbara's husband, John.

LESLIE GALLAGHER

Water Babies

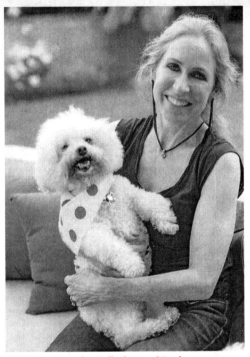

Leslie Gallagher and Pooh.

eslie Gallagher is the founder and director of Two Hands Four Paws, a rehabilitation center for animals in Santa Monica, California, that specializes in physical therapy. Tall, slender, and athletic—she runs five miles a day—Leslie grew up on an unusual farm in Stockton, in Northern California. Her father, an obstetrician and gynecologist, would come home from the hospital every day at five or six o'clock and hop on the tractor and till the fields until it was dark. Her mother taught English as a second language and looked after a full house: Leslie's brother and sister, as well as some children of Mexican farm laborers who came to Stockton each year to pick the crops.

"We grew every crop you could imagine—corn, potatoes, cauliflower—and cultivated at least twenty different kinds of fruit trees. We had so much produce, in fact, that we ended up feeding half the neighborhood. We baked our own bread and made our own ice cream. The rule was we don't buy any food at the grocery store that we can grow ourselves.

"It sounds more idyllic than it was," Leslie says. "My parents' marriage was unhappy, and I was keenly aware of it."

But when she was thirteen and got her first horse, Watusi, her whole life suddenly changed. "Watusi was a barrel racer and pigeon-toed. His owner had fallen on hard times and was no longer able to take care of him. My father saw the ad in the paper and we went to have a look. He was a bay with stunning light blue eyes and black hair, and there was something very special about him. I loved him the minute I set eyes on him. I loved that horse more than any other animal I'd ever lived with.

"We had an instant connection. We'd ride for hours and hours through cherry orchards, cornfields, and bean fields. I learned to file his hooves on the inside to keep him from tripping. At night when my parents had one of their horrific fights, I would go to the barn and sleep next to Wattie. The barn, the dogs, and Wattie (Watusi) were my refuge."

Leslie had to leave Wattie behind when she went off to boarding school in Connecticut. One night in her first year, she had a strange and upsetting dream. "I woke and told my roommate I had a nightmare that Wattie had died."

Her roommate suggested she call her parents, but Leslie figured if anything happened to her horse, they'd call her. She remembers, "But for the next week, I felt a terrible sadness.

"Then, my sister called. 'Are you sitting down?' she asked.

"A sick feeling rose in the pit of my stomach. My sister had gone to our parents' home in Stockton and learned that Wattie died. He'd had a stroke and wasn't able to get up on his legs. The veterinarian had to shoot him. My screams must have been heard all over Connecticut.

"If this happened today," Leslie stresses, "I would have taken him to UC Davis or to the nearest veterinary hospital that has physical therapy and gotten him onto an underwater treadmill for horses."

❧

Leslie went on to Scripps College, where she got a degree in international relations and was hired as Director of International Affairs for a foreign-based media mogul. He died and left behind an aging German shepherd, Sophie, that Leslie adored. She wound up adopting her.

A few months later there was an accident: a groomer dropped Sophie in the tub; as a result, the dog was left paralyzed. "I took her to surgeons, chiropractors, homeopaths—no one could do anything to help her," Leslie recalls. "I was so angry that there was nobody in Los Angeles who knew anything about doing physical therapy on dogs! Then my brother's wife suggested 'swimming' her. Within four weeks, I had her walking again."

That decided her. At thirty-five, Leslie embarked on a second career. She went back to school to earn degrees in canine and human massage therapy and canine rehabilitation. At the same time, she volunteered in the office of a board-certified veterinary surgeon to get a feel for the cases she might be taking on.

Then, using her savings from her previous job, she launched her own animal rehabilitation business out of her garage, with a pop-up pool and a treadmill. "I hung up my shingle and started getting dog after dog after dog," she recalls.

In just a few years, Leslie was able to expand to a six-thousand-square-foot facility with a state-of-the-art, thirty-foot pool, customized underwater and land treadmills, and acupuncture and laser-therapy programs. She now oversees a team of twenty-five veterinarians, acupuncturists, and certified therapists who treat about forty dogs a day.

Of the many dogs that had to be brought into the clinic on stretchers, one of the most challenging was an abandoned Doberman named Kenny, paralyzed after a metal door was dropped on his neck. Leslie met with her team and worked out a rigorous program that included swimming, massage, laser therapy, acupuncture, and assisted standing and walking. After surgery (paid for by donations) and many, many months of intense rehab, Kenny was able to run and jump, and play like any other dog. His against-all-odds recovery was videoed and picked up by media outlets around the world.

Leslie is frustrated that so many veterinarians are still not on board with physical therapy. A prominent older veterinary surgeon told her, "We've been practicing good medicine the same way for forty years. Why should we change now? I love you, I think you're great. If I believed in physical therapy, I would send you clients. But I don't really believe in it."

Leslie argues that if they just look at human studies they would see that as soon as a patient is cleared by a doctor, nearly every single person with a new hip or knee gets into the pool and works with a physical therapist. "When my husband had his knee replaced, we had a home nurse every single day for physical therapy. You can't refute the years and years of the science behind the fact that physical therapy helps people. Why not extrapolate that to animals?

"'You may be right," that eminent vet said, 'but it's not in my frame of reference.'"

Leslie says that attitude drove her wild, and so for years she went from hospital to hospital giving lectures and talking to veterinarians and their support staff about what they do at Two Hands Four Paws.

Leslie feels that one of her crowning achievements is having Dr. Stephen Ettinger, famous for his textbooks on veterinary internal medicine, as her Medical Director. She was honored that a veterinarian with his level of knowledge and expertise wanted to work with her. Eventually, Leslie convinced him to write about physical therapy. Consequently, the next edition of *Veterinary Internal Medicine* will cover animal rehabilitation. Leslie says it is her legacy; every veterinarian in the world will now study and learn about physical therapy.

She agonizes over how many people she comes across who don't want to care for or even live with a paralyzed dog. A story close to her heart is of a three-month-old golden retriever. It started with a phone call from a veterinary hospital telling her they had a puppy that was paralyzed in all four legs

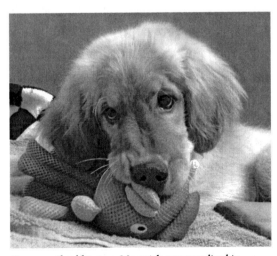

Four-month-old puppy, Maverick, was paralyzed in all four legs and was sheduled for euthanisia.

as a result of a freak reaction to a vaccine. The puppy's owners were about to euthanize him. Leslie says she went berserk. She got in touch with the owners immediately and lobbied to have Maverick given to her so she could take a shot at trying to get him walking again.

Six weeks went by, Leslie calling repeatedly to check on the puppy. "When an animal becomes paralyzed, every hour that goes by is crucial; you have between six to eight hours to get them in for an MRI and surgery, (if necessary) to try to reverse the damage. Sometimes waiting even twenty-four hours is too long because muscles can begin to atrophy and lose flexibility, which is often irreversible."

Finally, the hospital manager called Leslie. Maverick's owners decided *not* to euthanize. They were going to bring him to her.

"Maverick, the paralyzed puppy, entered my life.

"In the time that he was in the hospital, Maverick had not gotten any better; in fact, he was dramatically worse. He could not bend a single joint. He couldn't even move. Not a single joint, tendon, ligament, muscle, or body part worked on this dog. Even his eyelids were paralyzed! Every single joint needed correcting. Nothing moved in the right direction! I sat with Maverick and tried to figure out what I could do for him.

"We tried the underwater treadmill, but that was a challenge because none of his legs worked. So we tried suspending him from cables, with one person in the front working on his front legs and another person in the back working the hind legs. It was tight quarters with two people and a squirming puppy; we decided it would be smarter to get him in the water in the pool, where people could be in there with him.

LESLIE GALLAGHER

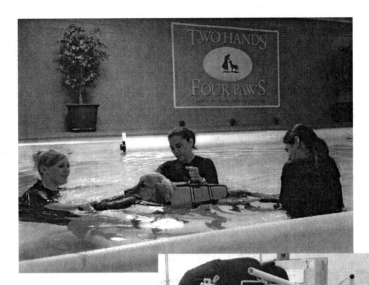

Above: Maverick in the big pool in a float coat.

Right: Using suspension in the underwater treadmill.

"We put a float coat on him and started with four people, one person sort of steering him around the pool, one working the front legs, another working the back legs, and one holding treats in front of him to try to get him to go forward. It was challenging because not only did his legs not work, but they were starting to grow twisted in the wrong direction. In some cases, they were growing sideways, and in one case, backwards. It wasn't two hands and four paws at that point; it took eight hands and four paws to pattern his legs in a normal gait.

"When you have a completely paralyzed dog getting in the water, they're going to be terrified, regardless of whether they're a swimming breed or not. If you let go of them or if they don't have a float coat on, they're going to hit the bottom of the pool. We used all kinds of squeaky toys and tennis balls to hold his interest. And he was much better if there was another dog in the pool because he really likes the company of other dogs.

"Three months went by, with therapists spending hours each day stretching and massaging Maverick's twisted limbs, using electrical stimulation on his muscles to try to kick-start them back to life, along with acupuncture and everything we had to get him walking again."

And then one day it happened. Leslie and her crew were working on Maverick, stretching his limbs to mimic the motions of standing and walking, when all of a sudden he wobbled to his feet. Leslie says it was suddenly so quiet, you could have heard a pin drop. "Then, bursting with excitement, everyone was laughing and screaming... Maverick with such a look on his face—a smile as big as the moon, his tail wagging furiously. Everyone cheered and clapped as they stood around the grinning puppy.

"And then he fell down. It was one of those moments that takes your breath away. And then, he did it again. Wobbling like mad, he struggled to his feet. The therapy was working! At last.

"The next day, Maverick took his first step. The only problem was that he could only walk backwards! For some reason, walking backwards seemed to come more naturally, or maybe just easier for him. Being able to stand and take a few steps backwards was a huge accomplishment."

Leslie noticed that taking even a few steps winded him. She realized he had absolutely no cardio fitness, which made sense because he hadn't moved in months. She thought his lungs probably hadn't developed normally and what little cardio fitness he'd had was gone. Maverick needed more time in the pool. Leslie and her team had to build his strength and muscle mass and, most importantly, get his lungs working.

"My even bigger concern, now that he was starting to move," Leslie says, "was that he *not* learn to walk incorrectly. This became a stressful catch-22. He *had* to learn to walk, bear weight, build muscle mass, and improve his cardio fitness. But he couldn't do it the wrong way."

Once again, Leslie and her team had to campaign for donations, this time using social media. People came forward, Maverick had one surgery to correct his deformed legs. After surgery, he had physical therapy every day for about a year. Leslie reports that today, "He's walking and running. He can even gallop. I mean, it's not pretty; you would never put him in Westminster, but he's a really sweet puppy and a complete goofball. I would place him if I could find a great home for him.

"For us, putting an animal in water can be magic. Swimming is the most powerful modality that we have with dogs who've had a stroke, for instance. The action of swimming and paddling the legs through the water actually clears the neural pathways and allows, for example, a clot in the spine to get out of the way of the nerves so that the nerves can start functioning again. With some of these stroke dogs, once we get them into the pool they often have quite a quick response—the pool seems to be pretty miraculous. In general, when you're creaky, when you're old, when your joints hurt, just floating in warm water and sometimes having jets going on painful joints feels so good to them."

Leslie describes the equally miraculous effects of the pool on horses. "The underwater treadmill, designed first for racehorses that incurred all kinds of injuries, was invented by one of the veterinarians who taught at my rehab school. Which is how the whole field of physical therapy for dogs started. And it worked so well for racehorses that therapists decided to adapt the underwater treadmill for dogs. That was how the field of canine rehab began. Today, animal rehabilitation is one of the fastest-growing areas in veterinary medicine.

"In our business we face a constant struggle of getting paralyzed dogs to walk again. Some owners and many vets give an animal very little time before announcing that a 'tough decision' has to be made. It's insanely frustrating because we know that, statistically, eighty percent of all paralyzed dogs will walk again. I remember years ago my very own vet (who obviously isn't my vet anymore) told me that he thought "down dogs" should be euthanized. I was blown away. I kept thinking of the dozens upon dozens of dogs I've seen over the years that were insanely happy running around in their wheelchairs."

❧

Leslie Gallagher gets emotional when she talks about animal rights. An outspoken activist, she feels strongly that animals have just as many rights in this world as people do, but they seem to get short shrift in life, especially those that live in countries other than the United States. "They're horribly mistreated. And even in our country, considering how much animals contribute to our well-being and happiness, so many are undervalued and underappreciated. I can't tell you how many times I've had people ask, especially on social media, *Why are you wasting your time and your energy on animals? Why don't you help people instead?* That just lights my hair on fire because people have resources and can pick up the phone and can get any help they need. An animal has no voice.

"I have animals come in here that are in excruciating pain and their owners don't even realize it. Then when we put them on some medication and do some therapy, the owner tells me, "'Oh my God. I had no idea how bad it was. He's so much better now.'

"These animals don't have a voice! It is my mission to spend every single day of my life trying to help them have a better quality of life, and to educate their caretakers about what we can do to make their lives better. These animals are so full of unconditional love, they will give their lives for us. We don't always appreciate that.

"We don't necessarily need to euthanize animals because they're sick or injured or disabled, not when there's so much we can do to help them. We must not give up on our animals! They are so faithful and so innocent and so needful of our love and our support. Let's do everything in our power to help them. I tell that to my clients every day. I'm willing to turn myself inside out and backwards and go the extra mile.

"If there aren't people like me out there fighting for them, fighting for their rights, and fighting to give them a better life, what hope is there for them?"

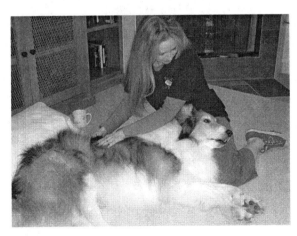

Bumper getting a massage.

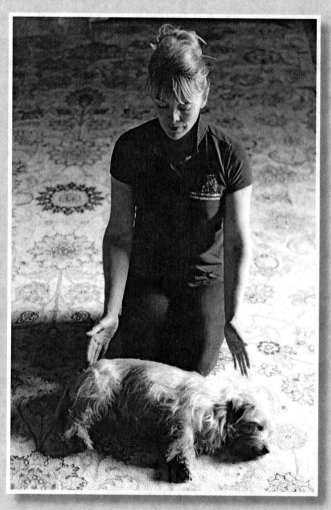

Elizabeth Whiter giving energy healing to Morris. Note: This photo also appears on the cover. PHOTO: Brian Clifford.

ELIZABETH WHITER

Pegasus

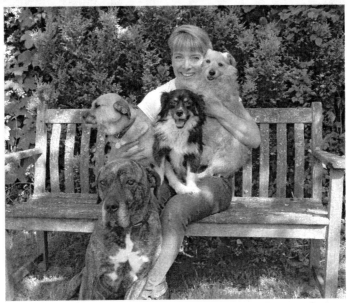

Elizabeth with her menagerie of rescue dogs. PHOTO: Brian Clifford.

𝓔lizabeth is a dynamo. Her large old rambling house, nestled in the South Downs National Park, Sussex, which is also her clinic, bustles with four rescue dogs, a cat, and just outside her office window, four horses, one of which was a national show jumper. The horses graze contentedly on eight acres. At the far end of the field near the stables are Elizabeth's herb gardens, which she calls her apothecary. Two of Elizabeth's assistants pop in and out of her office bringing patient files or in search of papers, telephones ring, a fax buzzes. Elizabeth speaks enthusiastically in her very West Country British accent, her voice frequently filled with passion about her work.

Born in London, raised in Somerset, Elizabeth developed her love of horses early. At seven she was riding; by the age of nine she was competing. Throughout her childhood and adolescence right up until she graduated from school, her bond with her horse was central to her life. She had intended to go to the University but got sidetracked and went straight into publishing at Haymarket Publishing, then the *Daily Mail,* a national newspaper where she set up a news section that was highly successful. Best of all, she was able to move her horse to the city with her.

After a two-year marriage that ended in divorce, Elizabeth became disenchanted with London. Her self-esteem bottomed out, she needed to be back in nature. She moved back to Somerset and she met her second husband, Brian.

When Brian Clifford came into her life and at the same time, "a beautiful horse, a seven-year-old grey gelding show jumper named Wow showed up," Elizabeth felt doubly blessed. "Wow was a super horse, a 'Pegasus,' who was kind and gentle and loved to go on trail rides through the countryside and enjoy nature. He also had a love for jumping big fences." Of the several animals in their household, Wow held a special place in her heart. Her life had turned around at last. Or so it seemed.

One autumn night soon after she and Brian were married, a sudden freak storm rose up, bringing deafening cracks of lightning and crashing thunder. Wow was in the paddock next to the house for the night, his rug securely fastened around him. When the storm broke, the terrified horse jumped the five-foot gate and tore off down the lane. A neighbor's swimming pool was covered with a canvas; unable to see it, Wow tumbled into the pool. The water-saturated rug weighed him down, but still he managed to scramble out of the pool and make his way back to Elizabeth's fields.

"That next morning, I found him standing there, bruised and scratched. We had no idea what had happened to him, nobody saw it happen. I called the vet immediately. After examining Wow carefully, he treated him for shock and thought that was the end of it. But over the next six months, even with the vet coming out repeatedly to check him, it was clear that Wow was deteriorating.

"Another vet came out to attend to Betty, my beautiful mare. At the stable door, he paused. 'Who is this chap here?'

"'This is Wow.' And I burst into tears. 'I don't know what's the matter with him, but you know, he's not happy. He had this terrible accident with a swimming pool,' I said, and explained what happened.

"'I have just recently become involved with equine osteopathy,' he said, 'and I'm training with Anthony Pusey, who works with the Queen and her horses. The Queen is very interested in equine osteopathy.' He suggested that we take him to the Animal Trust near Cambridge where they could do a scintigraphy scan—similar to an MRI."

The scan showed that Wow's neck was broken in three places. The prognosis was poor. The head technician came out to talk to Elizabeth. "I cannot see a way forward for your horse."

The meaning was clear.

"That night I sat with him in his stable, devastated. After a while I stood and walked around him, stroking him gently and whispering words of love and comfort. Suddenly, I felt compelled to place my hands on the broken places in his body, and right away I saw something change. He sighed, his eyes grew soft and relaxed and there was a shift in his energy. His head came down and he kissed me with his body language. Then by putting his head on my neck and moving me to where he wanted me to be, he ushered me around to his back. My horse was guiding me! My hands began to tingle as I realized that there were parts of his body that were cooler, and some parts were actually hot. Wow was teaching me!

"I felt our hearts connect in pure unconditional love. It was more than love; more than an emotional attachment, it was a magnetic force of energy. Wow's muscles began to quiver, his back legs started to relax, and I could see that he was processing, releasing. We got into a rhythm with our breaths, breathing deeper and deeper in unison. And then, he dropped off to sleep. When he woke he nodded his head as if to say, 'Thank you. I've had enough. I need space now.' And he walked to the back of the stable. He needed time to process.

"I didn't know what I was doing at that stage. I had never done any healing; I didn't even know anything about healing. I felt like crying with joy, seeing my horse so relaxed. Wondering if it could happen again, I went back the next night and did the same thing, staying very grounded, very centered, and focusing on sending him unconditional love. Wow responded exactly the same way. This is just incredible, I thought. Something important is happening and I have to know more about it."

Elizabeth called the new vet and told him what the scintigraph had shown and what the prognosis was. "I want you to come to the clinic with Wow," he said, "and meet Tony Pusey. We're going to have an osteopathy treatment with him."

Her eyes filled with tears of gratitude. At last an answered prayer. Elizabeth knew deep down that this was the person who could help Wow. She counted the minutes till the appointed day.

ELIZABETH WHITER

"Pusey was strapped into a body protector suit that made him look like the Michelin Man. He waddled over to Wow's stable and for the next half hour he manipulated the bones in Wow's spine. He was amazed at how calm and relaxed the horse was. Usually, he said, with a new patient he would have to administer a local anesthetic. I explained what I'd been doing each day, and he said that it had the same effect as an anesthetic. He confirmed that indeed Wow had suffered three severe breaks in his neck. He'd never seen anything that bad; he was lucky to be alive. I realized then how powerful my sessions with Wow were.

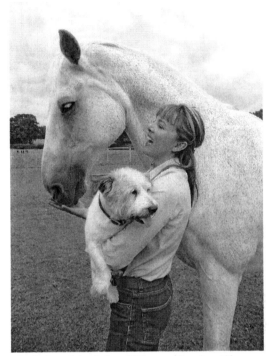

Elizabeth with her beloved Wow, and her dog, Alf.
PHOTO: Brian Clifford.

"Over the next year Wow continued to receive osteopathy treatments with Tony and I continued to have my private sessions with him as well. Witnessing Wow's improvement with osteopathy and his receptiveness and response to me transformed my life. I began to look into other complementary therapies: nutrition, kinesiology, energy healing, and zoopharmacognosy (from the Greek: zoo (animal), pharma (drug), and gnosy (knowing)).

"I first became aware of zoopharmacognosy, an animal's self-selecting process, when I discovered Wow eating the bark of a willow tree. None of my horses had ever done that, and I wondered then if he was doing some form of self-medication. I looked it up: Willow tree, I learned, is salicylic acid, which is what aspirin is made from. He was self-medicating for pain! Then I noticed he was also eating rose hips for Vitamin C and bladderwrack for electrolytes, all of which help repair the body.

"I decided I had to take the eight-year training in all the healing disciplines that were being offered by various accredited colleges in the UK. I wanted to establish myself as a professional

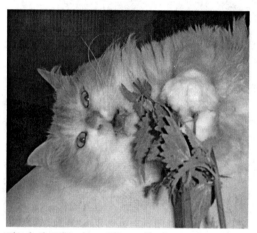

Elizabeth Whiter's cat Oliver self-selecting Catnip
Nepeta cataria.

and insured animal and human complementary therapist. I was particularly fond of the Healing Trust, which is the largest official healing organization in the UK. I studied there for two years, and then went on to the Ingraham Academy to study Zoopharmacognosy for three years, and I took intuition and insight classes at the London College of Psychic Studies, too.

"I traveled to South Africa to work with Jane Goodall and her primates, and a variety of wild animals such as cheetahs and lions; then on to Animal Care in Egypt, the equine and donkey hospital, to assist vets; and to Japan to work at animal outreach projects."

By 2000, Elizabeth was ready to open a healing center in her own house. Other healers, complementary therapists, animal professionals, and even vets joined her and together they worked with any and all animals, including bats, birds, and snakes.

In 2005, she established her animal training facility, the Healing Animals Organisation, where students from around the world, including veterinarians, can attend lectures, and workshops, and enroll in her diploma courses. Articles began to appear in several newspapers and she was being invited to appear on BBC and speak at colleges and wildlife charities worldwide.

"We became one of the only organizations in the United Kingdom that offers a two-year healing course for animals and their human guardians as well." Currently, there are four hundred graduates all over the world who have completed her training, and many of her students and graduates join her every year to offer healing and complementary rehabilitation skills at animal charities in the UK, Cyprus, Sri Lanka, Egypt, South Africa and many other parts of Europe.

Elizabeth has written two books: *The Animal Healer* (Hay House 2009), a number one best seller on Amazon, and *You Can Heal Your Pet: The Practical Guide to Holistic Health and Veterinary Care* (Hay House 2015), with Dr. Rohini Sathish, an integrative veterinary surgeon.

❧

Wow made a full recovery and lived to be twenty-three years old. Right up until his passing, Wow was one of the principal teachers for Elizabeth's Diploma in Equine Healing, and a key player. In Elizabeth's human clinic, horses are also healers, helping patients of all age groups to find confidence and self-awareness.

Elizabeth credits Wow with changing her life; he was her greatest teacher. From him she feels she learned the true meaning of unconditional love.

❧ ❧ ❧

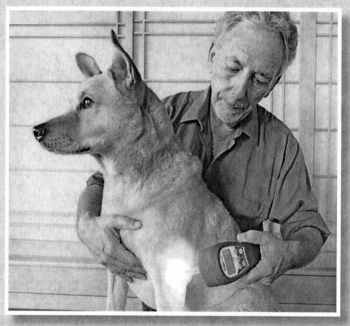

Therapeutic use of ACTIVet Pro low level laser for the treatment of elbow arthritis in a dog.
Photo: J. Mark Strong, Director, Global Development, Multiradiance Medical.

ALLEN MARK SCHOEN,
DVM, MS, PH.D. (HON.)

The Middle Path

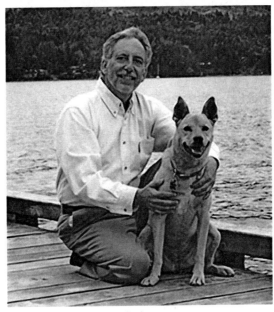

Kindred spirits.

$\mathcal{F}$amed trailblazer in the world of veterinary medicine, Dr. Allen Schoen has managed to bridge the gap between conventional and alternative therapies. After earning multiple advanced degrees—DVM from Cornell University, a master's in neurophysiology and animal behavior from the University of Illinois—he discovered that his real interest, his *passion*, was to find out what he could do for animals that did not respond to conventional medicine. He studied acupuncture, which, he felt, was really applied neurophysiology and neuroimmunology. "From then on, I have always danced between science and energy healing, integrating them wherever I could."

Even as a young boy, Allen knew he wanted to be an animal doctor. In English class, everything he wrote about was animals and how to help them. "Even though we didn't have pets at home—my parents were immigrants who were just trying to survive—still, they put up with my obsession. In high school, except for biology class, I found myself bored, so the summer between my junior and senior year, I applied for a biology program at the University of Bridgeport in Connecticut run by Dr. Eugene Somers that was like a biology boot camp. My dream was to go to Cornell University, known at the time for having the best veterinary school in the world. Dr. Somers became one of my greatest mentors. At the end of the summer, knowing I was contemplating dropping out of high school, Dr. Somers offered me the opportunity to study biology under his tutelage there at the university. When I told him that my parents did not have the money to send me to college, he offered me a full scholarship—as long as I kept up my grades. That catapulted me into high gear; it was an important validation of my passionate love of biology. Following my heart actually worked!

"Animal behavior and the study of consciousness were my other passions. I ended up applying to veterinary schools, and a few graduate programs in animal behavior. I chose to pursue a master's degree in animal behavior at the University of Illinois. My commitment was never to do any research that would harm animals.

"My dream of going to Cornell University College of Veterinary Medicine was realized, too. But despite being the greatest vet school providing the best education in conventional medicine and surgery, it was limited to medicine and surgery. What I felt was missing, what was being shut down in me, was this heart connection—the very reason that I went into veterinary medicine."

Following a few years of practicing, Allen's passion to help animals that could not be helped in any conventional way led him to expand his knowledge by studying acupuncture, Chinese herbs, Western herbs, chiropractic, nutrition, and the human-animal bond.

In 1982, he launched the Department of Acupuncture at the Animal Medical Center in NYC. It was the first department of veterinary acupuncture outside of China, and at the largest animal hospital in the world.

Allen went on to become a clinical assistant professor teaching integrative medicine at both Colorado State University College of Veterinary Medicine & Biomedical Sciences and at Tufts University. He also served on a committee for the American Veterinary Medical Association to develop guidelines for alternative medicine, all while continuing his integrative vet practice in Connecticut and New York.

"The way I was able to bridge the gap between the disciplines was by seeing that there was no real difference between the two, just a matter of understanding the various perspectives on healing.

"There is a place for everything. A number of holistic veterinarians and practitioners seem to have a chip on their shoulders, claiming that all Western medicine is bad and that only holistic medicine works. At the other extreme, many conventional veterinarians claim that holistic and alternative medicine is quackery, and that only drugs and surgery work. I believe reality lies somewhere in the middle. There's certainly a place for medicine and surgery. There's a place for vaccines too, but we seem to have sometimes gone to extremes there as well. With the development and availability of so many vaccines, there is the potential to over-stimulate the immune system, which may result in immune-mediated disorders. For years, veterinarians said that dogs and cats need vaccines every year; now it has been shown that most vaccines may last for years. A safer way to protect animals from infectious diseases may be to use blood tests that evaluate the blood titer, the level of antibodies that protects against specific diseases. Legally, some animals need a rabies vaccination periodically. With antibiotics, I've seen instances where they are the best option; however, there are other antibacterial and antimicrobial agents that may be beneficial if the animal is not in crisis. It's not unreasonable to try those first in appropriate situations. The increase in antibiotic resistance may be due in part to the heavy use of antibiotics in food-producing animals.

"I try to bring some balance to all these concerns, because I do see so many animals suffer adverse reactions to vaccines, effects that conventional veterinarians might not associate with vaccinations. Whenever I am consulting on a chronic condition in an animal, I ask: When did the problems first start, and what happened in the weeks and months beforehand? If a vaccination preceded the condition, I ask: How soon after that did you see reactions? Whether it's considered coincidental or not depends upon whom you talk to, but note how often immune-mediated disorders will follow shortly after a series of vaccinations. Of course, that doesn't happen with every animal, but it happens enough that we need to be aware of the possibility. In addition, if you read the fine print on vaccines, it always says they should be given only to healthy animals. What is a healthy animal, and how often are those vaccines given to animals that are not in a state of health? My attitude is judicious use. You weigh the pros and cons, the risks and benefits, whether conventional or complementary or holistic. It is much like the 'Middle Path' of Buddhist practice."

ALLEN MARK SCHOEN

Before long, Dr. Schoen became known as one of the leading authorities on holistic, integrative medicine, and was in great demand as a speaker and lecturer. The heads of internal medicine, surgery, neurosurgery, and radiology at the Animal Medical Center in New York invited him to give a lecture on the scientific basis of acupuncture. "At the end of that lecture, the head of neurosurgery came up to me and said, 'I am going to do everything I can to make sure you're not here.' But the head of the Medical Center disagreed. He offered to set up a study of acupuncture at the Center, stating that, 'If we feel that Western medicine and surgery have failed with an animal and we're recommending euthanasia, we'll refer them to you.'

"It seemed like the closest possibility of a controlled clinical trial. I didn't take on all the cases. I accepted only those patients for whom I felt acupuncture would be beneficial. Of the animals that I chose to treat, eighty percent were able to live longer, healthier, happier, pain-free lives. Each one of those animals had been recommended for euthanasia.

"Those successes served to eliminate the placebo effect from the equation, which was the major argument against acupuncture. At conferences (about human patients) where I was invited to lecture, I explained that when you see acupuncture work for animals, you realize it cannot be a placebo. By documenting cases well, I was able to show that a significant number of animals that were not responding to medicine and surgery and were earmarked for euthanasia, did respond to acupuncture.

"There are many other advances in veterinary medicine now such as low-level laser therapy," Allen explains. "The use of light energy, of low-level lasers, can help heal the body by increasing microcirculation. Electro-acupuncture, therapeutic ultrasound, and pulsed electromagnetic fields have all expanded a great deal since thirty years ago when veterinary medicine was limited to medications and surgery.

"We still have a long way to go. Twenty years ago, I took training in medical Qigong, and started integrating that discipline into my veterinary practices. There are many different ancient Eastern traditions of energy healing, from medical Qigong to Reiki and numerous others. We may still not have a thorough understanding and appreciation of their mechanism of action. Part of my journey has been to try to better understand the scientific basis of various healing modalities, but sometimes those elements defy our current limited understanding. So many approaches that were not acknowledged during my veterinary school training are now better understood and have been integrated into current veterinary medicine.

"Everything is energy. In my new book, *The Compassionate Equestrian* (Trafalgar Books, June 2015), I discuss my two new theories. One I call the Transspecies Field Theory, which is based on quantum physics, neuroscience, HeartMath, and other explorations. I describe that an energetic field is created between all the animals with which we interact. For example, how often do we go into a horse barn and immediately feel an uncomfortable or angry energy? The horses' ears are back, they're not happy, the grooms aren't happy, no one seems happy. But then you might go into another horse barn where everyone's singing and pleasant, humans and animals alike are relaxed and happy. Or we go to an animal hospital and sense an uneasy or anxious feeling and think, 'Oh God, get me out of this one,' whereas in another hospital or animal shelter we sense a feeling of peace and a wonderful energy that has the opposite effect.

"And then I also propose that when we put forth an intention of compassion, we can actually have a positive impact on the field, rather than being just an unconscious part of it; and we can change the field to be a happier, healthier, and more loving field.

"One hears more and more about the healing benefits of therapeutic touch. I have my own terms for it. I put my hands on the animals and do what I call a pet scan. My pet scan integrates a conventional physical examination—palpating an animal all over—along with feeling certain acupuncture points for any sensitivity that may relate to internal organs or different acupuncture pathways. While I'm palpating the animal, the energy that is exchanged may be therapeutic as well.

"I am sometimes asked if I am an animal communicator. My answer is that we are *all* animal communicators; all we have to do is be open to the awareness that we are. Animals are communicating with us all the time, it just happens at different levels. It is we who block that communication. Like anything else, it's where we put our intention, our awareness, and our energy.

"As a veterinarian and scientist, I used to have a certain skepticism about distance healing, but having on occasion seen its effectiveness firsthand, I felt a need to open my mind more and explore the ways in which it might be possible. I realized that only through having some appreciation of quantum physics can one even try to explain the phenomenon. That is one of my other passions. If you say you understand quantum physics, you don't—so I certainly don't say I can understand it, but I am fascinated. It does provide some explanation for certain effects that are beyond our comprehension, like the gift of healers who have the sensitivity and the training to be of great benefit to animals."

On the subject of cancer treatments, Allen explains he has to leave the choice to his clients. "I find that if clients have had good success or improvement with chemotherapy or radiation for themselves or a relative, then they believe in it. If they've had negative experiences and decide they don't want to go in that direction, I try a more holistic, integrative approach. I might suggest a consultation with an integrative oncologist. With chemotherapy and radiation therapy, it's always important to ask what are the risks involved, what are the successes, and what are the potential side effects. I always tell clients, 'Once you have consulted with an oncologist, come back to me, and based on your choice, we will develop a complementary approach. If you choose not to go for chemotherapy or radiation, then we can treat more holistically. If you choose chemotherapy or radiation, I'll add some approaches that minimize the side effects and that can help to rebuild the body afterwards.' It would be detrimental to someone who believes in a particular approach to shatter that belief. So, I try to offer my clients a bouquet of different therapies and see which combination is best suited to the client and their animal companion.

"Sometimes you sense that it's time for an animal to die, to let go. Sometimes it seems as if it's the *people* who aren't ready to let go, and who feel that they have to do something more. In those situations, I'll offer some palliative care to help relieve the animal's pain and suffering. It perturbs me when I see a veterinarian recommend different types of chemotherapy or radiation treatments that may not have the data or the success rate behind them. Yet, because the client is not ready to let go, they suggest more potentially toxic approaches that may cause the animal even more pain and suffering. It always goes back to the spirit of our Hippocratic Oath: First, do no harm. This is always uppermost in my mind.

"One of the reasons I was successful in opening the doors of veterinary medicine to understanding that there is more to healing than just medications and surgery was my respect for conventional medicine while at the same time acknowledging a more complementary approach. No one form of medicine has all the answers; a truly integrative approach is the key. There are healing mechanisms that go far beyond our current understanding of energy. We are all part of a greater consciousness, a greater energy that flows through us. My goal is to be of benefit to each animal as well as to that collective consciousness."

Allen Schoen's journey has not been without its hurdles. Throughout his career, he experienced resistance to some of his methods from extremist skeptics and cynics. He also went through some personal life challenges and transitions—divorce, the sale of most of his veterinary practice, and then the death of his cat Chi and his dog Shanti, both of old age. His time on the East Coast had come to an end; it was time to make a major move. "When I was six years old, growing up in a basement in Queens, I had actually circled an area in British Columbia on a map, declaring that someday I would live there. For years, I kept feeling that place calling to me. Then, in the late '90s, the Alberta and British Columbia Veterinary Medical Associations invited me to come west and train their veterinarians in acupuncture and natural medicine.

"Over dinner one night, one of the vets studying with me said, 'Allen, you know you belong here.' The next time I was in Vancouver teaching, I visited this small island and all of a sudden, I felt at home. Three days later, I came upon a cabin. It had the same view I saw when I was six years old! This was a mystery I had to pursue. If I didn't, I wouldn't be following the mystery of my life. Once I got that, it all started to unfold. I heard that still, inner voice telling me, *This is going to be a healing center, not just for you but for countless beings, and in countless ways that you have no conception of at this moment.* I kept being called to be here more and more. That's when I began to let go of my previous life back East. This cabin became my retreat where I do my writing and development of new approaches to healing."

Allen still travels back to the East Coast to Connecticut a few times a year where he gets into his old Jeep and drives around from barn-to-barn, seeing clients and patients, which is one of the reasons he kept putting off having pets of his own. "Also, by not having a dog or a cat, a Garden of Eden has shown up here. Two families of deer were born under my deck each year—one had twins. And as soon as they were born the mothers brought them to my front door. I have shared these years with four or five generations of them. They just come, look in the windows, and lie down by the front door and hang out. They've even run into the house. I had to catch them and take them outside. Eagles, hummingbirds, numerous seabirds, loons—all live here year-round and we share our lives and this space together. Some mornings I wake to see an eagle sitting on the tree in front of my bedroom window, just looking in at me. Other days, the hummingbirds come to the window and peek in. And if I'm sitting out on my deck, they'll zip right in front of my eyes to look at me. Now, eagles and otters and seals all come. It truly is a Garden of Eden! Oddly enough, two months ago a pair of peacocks showed up. They roost in my neighbor's trees, but most mornings they come over here and hang out all day, watching and following me through the windows. If I'm sitting on the deck, they'll come over and lie down, one on either side of me.

"I think if I had my own dog and cat some of the wildlife might be scared away. What I realize is, wildlife feels safe here in this whole transspecies energetic field—the deer, the songbirds, the hummingbirds, and the peacocks. It's really quite amazing. My whole life was so goal-oriented, my passion always driving me to explore the next approach in healing. It seemed that just when I thought I got it all down, another animal would show up and I'd see that my current understanding of healing was insufficient. And that would inspire me to explore some new approach. It seems now that the wild animals are mainly showing me that we are all truly interconnected, and that it is only our programmed beliefs that limit what we see.

"Over the past fourteen years, I really needed to open my mind—and my heart—even more, and be increasingly receptive to what healing truly is. I understand now that creating silence and surrendering to the unfolding allows things to show up in my life that were once beyond my expectations and my understanding. I find that the more I broaden my perspective, the more I see showing up for me. And as more shows up for me, my beliefs expand further, as does my mind. I can appreciate even greater aspects of healing, healing that we don't even have labels for. That is why my journey has been—and will ever be—a quest for ultimate healing.

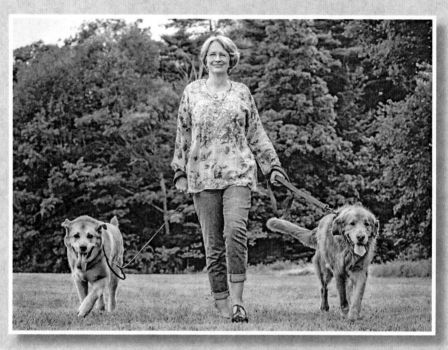

Bower and Smitty always enjoy a walk after a healing session.
Photo: Franco Vogt.

CINDY BRODY

CinergE

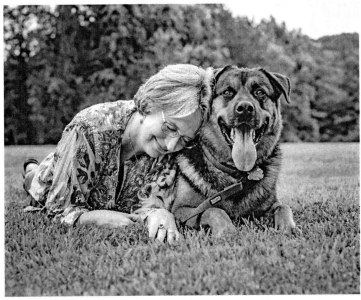

Through CinergE relationships grow. Communication and energy healing build bonds. PHOTO: Franco Vogt.

"My goal is to help people and their animals understand each other and deepen their connection." CinergE is an energetic healing modality that Cindy Brody created. It combines her training as a Reiki Master with her intuitive skills as a healer that together encourage the body's own healing power. CinergE incorporates an array of complementary therapies such as energy balancing, muscle testing, Reiki, acupressure, intuition, and animal communication. The goal is to help relieve a sentient being's physical and mental stress, muscle tightness, and joint inflammation. Used together, these techniques unlock tension, promote healing, and boost the immune system.

When she was four years old, Cindy Brody discovered something wonderful about her young self. She had a dog named Fawn, a little guy of no particular breed that loved to play. But Fawn had a long back like a dachshund that was often sore and when it was, he stopped playing and would snap at her when she went to lift him. So Cindy would put her small hands gently on Fawn's back, and after a bit he would respond by eagerly wanting to play again.

On the farm in Nebraska where Cindy spent summers growing up, there were also cats and kittens that would often get sick. When they did, she would put her hands on them and close her eyes for several minutes until the kittens would begin to purr, become calm, and curl up and go to sleep. When her grandfather's dog became seriously ill, and her grandfather was beside himself with worry, Cindy placed her hands on the dog and the dog recovered.

And so it went: As she grew older, Cindy continued to put her hands on any of the animals that needed help and they always seemed to get better.

Cindy began to wonder what she had in her hands. Over ensuing years, she learned it was a form of "healing energy" that passed from her hands to animals. She came to name it Universal Life Energy. She believes everyone has the ability to channel it. Her imagery is that she takes this energy from the Universe, funneling it through the top of her head and then through her hands—always for a greater good.

In her early twenties, Cindy met people in the healing arts who used crystals to perform healings, and she was curious to try it. But she soon realized she didn't need crystals to amplify the energy in her hands, and would just feel the heat and use her intuition to focus on the images that came to her mind, showing her where the energy was blocked.

"I was living in New York City at the time. It was during the '80s when the AIDS epidemic was out of control and I was losing so many friends to it. I felt that I had to be working with people. I was in the restaurant business at the time in a very popular restaurant in New York, working as the maître d'. During service, whenever one of my waiters or waitresses had a meltdown, I would put my hands on them to calm them. But after a while, I started to burn out on the city and I decided to flee; I moved to Woodstock, New York. I had kids right away and then I started riding horses again.

"For twenty years I primarily worked with people, but all the while I was putting my hands on my own animals and healing them whenever necessary."

Soon Cindy began performing distance healing with people. She would ask the ailing person to send her something of a personal nature, such as hair from a hairbrush or even lint from clothing they liked to wear. She would then hold the item, meditate on it, and intuit what was needed to heal the individual. She discovered she could also use photographs with the same technique.

"My big life-changing aha moment came one day when I was in the barn and noticed that one of the horses I had been riding had gone lame. So, I placed my hands on her knee. My hands got really hot and she lowered her head and dropped her lip. I could hear her soft whinny as I worked on the other leg. I knew she had been coughing so I also put my hands on her chest.

"I didn't tell anybody what I was doing. The next time I came back to ride I heard someone commenting on how much better the horse was looking and how she wasn't limping or coughing as much. I thought, Woah, wait a minute. This is good! So, every time I returned to the barn after I rode I would stay and put my hands on the other horses. Again, this was not a barn that knew me; even to this day they don't know me. And they don't believe in the work. That was fine with me. Every time I put my hands on the horses, the same thing would happen. These animals have had a very hard life. They're older. They were once show horses; they've been running around in circles for most of their lives."

It was when Cindy learned how to use muscle testing—on people as well as animals—that her work as a healer truly blossomed. On horses, she was able to pinpoint exactly where the horse was holding tension, where it was injured, and where the blockages were that needed to be released. This technique complemented all the other tools she'd been using.

"At that point results were so obvious—surprising even—that soon people began to bring their dogs to the barn and I was treating everything from sore backs and lameness to Lyme disease and separation anxiety. Barn cats came in missing an eye, or limping. People would see me working on the animals and ask me if I would come to their house and help with their horse or their pet. And within a very short period of time, I was seeing anywhere from fifteen to thirty horses and dogs a week."

Cindy uses muscle testing to this day on horses to determine exactly where in their bodies they are experiencing tension or injury, and to relieve tension and open any energy blockages. She also learned Reiki, which she has incorporated into her healing practice, eventually becoming a teacher of Reiki.

CINDY BRODY

"I have been crazy about animals my whole life. There were times in my life when without them I would have been totally lost. My dogs have seen me through so many stages of my life, the loss of my mother as a child, hard times through my teens, and trying to find my way in a world that didn't always appreciate my 'special talents.' When I first became a mother, my sweet German Shorthaired Pointer, Molly, would lie on my feet for hours as I rocked my colicky baby. Molly was my lifeline. My dogs have always been there for me more than I can describe."

Using her intuition, Cindy has been able to "hear" animals. One example she gives is about a cat that lives in Oakland, California, with a woman who for twenty-three years fed a colony of stray cats. The woman would always have them neutered and spayed and provide them with a safe and loving haven. "This one particular cat, fourteen or fifteen years old, who had lived her whole life outdoors, suddenly became very ill. The woman took her to the vet, who diagnosed the cat with leukemia. She was told that the cat was going to pass away very soon.

"When the woman contacted me, I listened with my intuition for what the cat had to say. The first thing I understood was that she wanted to die as she'd lived, outside under a bush. 'I have a little bit of the taste of the wild in me,' she explained. I assumed that she was a feral cat.

"Soon after, the woman had to downsize, and she and her husband were forced to move. The new tenants promised they would continue to feed the cat, but even so the woman came back to the house every day to sit beside the dying cat. The woman asked me what she could do to help her. So, I gave her a very simple exercise to rub her hands together, feel the energy in them, and imagine the Universal Life Energy coming through the top of her head and down through her hands. 'Just place your hands on the cat's body.'

"There was a shift. The cat was now saying she loves to sit in this woman's lap. And the woman said that as soon as she puts her hands on the cat, the cat begins to purr and seems to be in a place of peace."

Cindy teaches people that what they do in the here and now can be life-changing. "Whether it's a dog that is depressed, a horse that bucks, or a cat that marks, each has a story. I give them a voice, and that helps to heal their bodies and souls. I speak to animals all over the country through long-distance animal communication. By looking into the animal's eyes in a photograph, I can help to bridge the communication gap between animals and humans, resolving issues that get in the way of training.

"My job is to help clear up misunderstandings, bring physical relief, and to teach people what we can do to help our four-legged family members have the best life possible. As a result, our lives improve. Every dog is a therapy dog, helping us by loving us unconditionally. Our problems often become their problems. We work too hard and come home stressed, we have our own physical pain or illness; they sense this and it can be quite upsetting for them. When we take better care of ourselves, they feel better too.

"When I work with dogs I find out what they are feeling, physically and mentally. As an animal communicator, I look into what the family dynamic is that feeds into the behavior. They will sometimes tell me that they are yelled at, or forced into a bedroom when visitors come. They often say that they want to be good dogs but they just don't know how. They don't understand why their people are so angry with them. The tone of your voice when you are calling a dog sends many messages.

"People need to bring me their dogs only once or twice. I give them tools that they can easily grasp, and I make it very simple so they can immediately start treating their own animals. I make sure to urge everybody I teach to share the program with any friend in need."

On her website, she suggests questions to ask your animal:

- How does your body feel? Does anything hurt?
- What are your favorite things to do?
- What are your least favorite things to do?
- Are you happy with your food?
- Is there anything you need?
- Do you have a message or advice for me?
- Do you like your kennel, pet sitter, trainer, walker, groomer...?
- Are you ready to pass over?
- Do you want a friend?

And questions for your horse:

- Are you in pain?
- How do your saddle, shoes, bit... fit?
- How are your neck, shoulders, back, hips, hocks...?
- Do you like your job?
- Do you have any advice for me in the way that I ride, train, etc.?
- Do you like your stall mate?
- What can I do to make your life easier?

It is now more than fifty years that Cindy Brody has been healing animals and people, working full time fifty to sixty hours a week. She also travels around the country teaching people how they can do the work themselves. Still, she manages to find time to work on her books.

Cindy lives in Woodstock, New York, with her husband and their son and daughter. She also has two grandchildren. She says she is living her dream.

❧ ❧ ❧

JAMES FRENCH

The Trust Technique

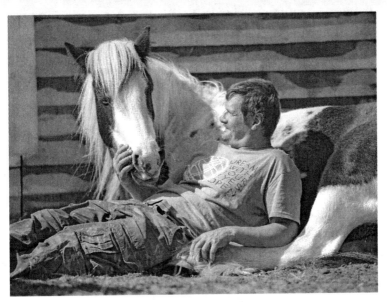

Bobbie and James share a relationship built on trust and nurture.
PHOTO: Brittany Sparham.

There are many stories of horse whisperers, but at Mane Chance Sanctuary in Surrey, England, the horses actually whisper back. Founded in 2011 by British actress Jenny Seagrove for the rescue of sick, abandoned, or abused horses, some are so emotionally damaged that Jenny called on renowned healer and communicator James French to work with them.

James is pioneer of the gentle but powerful approach he calls the Trust Technique. His sessions are quiet and still; he sits in a field with the animal (or if necessary, just outside the stall), empties his mind, and quietly contemplates the horse—or any animal—until gradually it grows calm and lies down next to him, often going to sleep. "It's about getting the limbic system—the part of the brain associated with emotions and memories—of horse and human in sync. The Trust Technique teaches mindfulness, how to let go of your own thinking."

James's rare gift grew out of an intensely traumatic childhood. Born in Hong Kong to a highly successful family in the fashion industry, he was just two years old when his family and several children, including his sister, went out on the family boat for a party. James had created a ruckus that morning and was made to stay at home with the nursemaid.

"That was the day of the accident. The petrol can in the boat fell over, causing a huge fire, and the boat burst into flames. Three children died, among them my sister. My dad was hospitalized, in traction, for eight months.

The family barely survived the tragedy. "We moved back to the UK, and soon after, my parents broke up and my mom and I moved to a farm. My mom, deep into grieving, surrounded herself with animals. I was literally brought up with seven dogs and three horses and a sheep. Before long, my mom invited into our lives a gentleman who was an angry alcoholic. Nobody but me, a seven-year-old, was aware that there was something very wrong. It was a very scary environment. My stepfather made three different attempts on my life, using axing tools and other scary things. I came to depend on the support of the animals around me, and out of need I developed a strong connection with them.

"It was my relationship with animals that saved me. I would go out and spend the whole day riding, just letting the horse take me. I never wanted any control over an animal; I didn't see them like that.

They were my relationships. If I wanted to go outside, no sooner did I have the thought then there'd be seven dogs right next to me and off we'd go. They'd always come and find me from wherever they were. As I grew into adulthood they were my only security.

"Time passed, my stepfather left, and I had to find work. Because I'd been riding since I was two-years-old, I decided I would go into the world of horses and work in all the disciplines from jumping to polo. I remember how appalled I was back then at the way the horses were treated.

"I started working with young horses, backing them—riding them for the first time. I was sent every horse that nobody else could back, including some really damaged horses, which is what forced me to find some completely new way to work. After observing the horses in their herds, I began to develop my own whispering technique, young as I was.

"One day, a lady, a chiropractor, came to see the horses that I was working with—she was a McTimoney chiropractor [a technique popular in the UK]. As she did her work, my hands were on the horses at the same time. She looked over at me. 'Did you know you're a healer?' I sort of smiled and nodded—I was only in my twenties. She invited me to come with her on her rounds and put my hands on the horses after she had worked on them. She would pay for the petrol.

"Suddenly I was being treated as a healer without really knowing how to describe what I was doing. Because if after I worked on a few horses the owner asked me what I was doing, I wouldn't know what to say. And of course, that moment did come. The word Reiki popped into my mind, a word I must have seen or heard somewhere, and that's what came out.

"Synchronicity. Two weeks later, I saw a friend from school whom I hadn't seen in a long time. We chatted and I asked him how his mum, whom I once knew really well, was doing. He told me she was a Reiki healer.

"I decided that's what I wanted to study. With my partner, Shelly, I studied first and second-degree Reiki. Once having learned it, I began to give the treatment to horses. But rather than working with them in the stall doing my whispering technique, I gave them Reiki until they were really peaceful, then I would put the tack on. If they came up in their mind at all, I would give them Reiki again until they were relaxed. Then I would climb on the horse in the stall. The only issue I had is that sometimes they were so relaxed it was hard to get them to move forward because they were asleep.

"For the next four years I studied for my mastership with lineage bearer Phyllis Lei Furumoto and traveled with her to Wales, Uruguay, and Australia. When she felt that I was ready, she invited me to come with her to Hawaii to be initiated. She was going to see her grandmother, an early Reiki master.

"After that, unusual things began to happen. While I was giving Reiki to horses and other animals, I found I was tuning in to their thoughts and feelings, picking up on what is known as animal communication. That opened up a completely different doorway for me. Not only was I administering a healing, I was also connecting to them and understanding what their upsets were. I believe I did that as a child, but it was so natural to me then that I wouldn't have recognized it as unusual.

"My first experience with animal communication was with a lovely old horse. As I put my hands on him and gave him Reiki, the horse communicated to me that his owner comes to him every night with the problem that she has in her stomach.

"At first I didn't really believe it; I dismissed it and carried on with the treatment. Then the communication came back to me again. 'The reason I've got this problem in my leg,' the old horse explained, 'is because of my owner's emotion. Because I look after her so much, her emotions got stuck in my leg.'

"I listened this time thinking, wow, this is very interesting. Okay, well, that's very deep, but what if it's all wrong? 'Could you just tell me something?' I asked. 'Something really simple that I can share with your lady?'

"The old horse told me he loved the grass she'd been giving him in his food. I looked at his bowl. You don't put grass in a horse's bowl, you put hog feed in there. I decided that when the lady came back, I'd share that little bit of information first, and if it turned out to be accurate, I'd tell her the rest.

"When she came back and asked how it went, I said rather sheepishly, 'Oh, he loves the grass you're giving him in his food.'

"'How did you know that? I've just started giving him dried grass food supplement in his food, and he loves it.'

"'Well, there's more information.' I shared that her horse felt she had a problem with her stomach.

"She burst into tears. 'Yes, for the past three years, my husband and I have been trying to have a baby. And just recently, it's gone so wrong, I've had to have a hysterectomy. And, yes, every evening I do go and see him. If that's what's making him ill, I feel so guilty.'

"Straight away, the old horse said, 'Oh, no, no, no. That's my job. It's my job to do this.'

"I then asked the horse what we could do to help him with his leg.

"'Well, I'm an old boy now,' he answered. 'But I used to do a lot of galloping. Both of us could do with a really good gallop.'

"And that was my recommendation for both of them, and that's what helped him to let go of the pain in his leg.

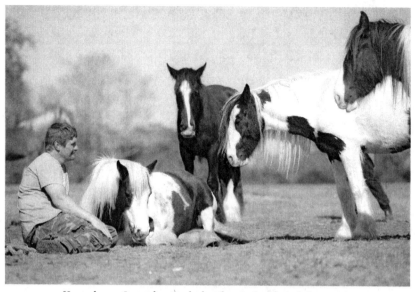

Young horses James has worked with enjoying their daily session.
PHOTO: Brittany Sparham.

"Something had opened up for me. My animal communication career had begun, and I was able to teach other people how to do it. It was really very easy. I would find out what the animal's problem was and then I would administer a healing. I discovered that animals and humans have a very detailed and shared relationship, and that animals are highly sensitive to how their people feel. Often the human is only reflecting what the animal feels, just as the animal is only reflecting what the human is feeling. The narratives of the animal and the human match, they are drawn to each other; it's the law of attraction. So, I can't just go in and mend an animal; I have to help the human as well.

"With these key elements, I discovered a way of breaking the reaction cycles: I created what I call the Trust Technique. It works by reducing the thinking levels of any type of animal so that their emotional state changes, allowing them to find confidence. It also teaches the human how to enter a relaxed and peaceful state of mind and how to deliver this peace of mind to the animal. This in turn creates a deeper relationship of trust and acts as a solid teaching foundation for the animal.

"It is a whole new level of interaction that works in unity with the emotions, and develops the spirit of the animal as well as the human.

"I have used this technique with horses, dogs, cats, and lions in South Africa, putting the two elements together in a very simple way that teaches people to do it for themselves and their animals. But it's developed even further. Shelly and I took over the management of the Mane Chance Sanctuary and created a project, a shared healing event. We take children, the ones who have real trouble at school—maybe they're on the autistic spectrum or have aggression issues—and teach them to be mindful with the horses. Damaged horses and damaged children work together, and in the process, each finds his or her self.

"One of the first horses I worked with at the sanctuary was Ernie, a massive horse of eighteen hands—if you're standing next to him as he walks past, the sun disappears. When I first saw Ernie, he was in a stable that was no bigger than he was, really, kept there 24/7 with a sign that read, 'I bite.' They referred to him as Dr. Death. Ernie had kicked one person in the head and sent him into a coma, and bitten another's cheek right off of his face, and someone else's fingers off. And he was never allowed to be with the other horses because he would pick them up and shake them like a rag doll.

"Ernie had been brought up by a farmer who was terrified of him and who took his anger out on the horse. Ernie learned fear aggression—to attack before he got hurt—from an early age. Jennie asked for our help.

"The first time I saw him was out in a field. I couldn't stay out there with him because he kept chasing me, so I had to work with him from outside his stall. Really all Ernie wanted was friendship. But he didn't understand about space, so he would come marching up to another horse and be very intimidating. Then, the moment he sensed fear he would attack. The same with people. There were stories of people trying to work with Ernie, and Ernie, sensing their fear, would strip their clothes right off their bodies.

"Ernie's communication to me was, 'I just want a friend.'

"I told him if he wanted a friend, he had to learn to be peaceful and wait for the friend to come to him.

"That was our first session. From then on, we had good communication. I was able to calm his mind until he actually fell asleep. Then I would take him out into the field. I chose the wisest horse in the park, a lovely horse named Barry, and putting a line in between their fields, I set a special time for them to be together. Big Ernie stood there and let Barry come to him. From there we advanced slowly until gradually Ernie understood, and he and Barry became great friends. That was three years ago when he was twenty-two. Now I have him go with Barry to meet the new horses we have coming to the site. Their very important role is to be the first to integrate with new horses.

"He's changed so much! This is a horse you couldn't put a head collar on or even handle; now anyone can groom him. He loves life. He's also valuable when we're working with kids, showing them to be peaceful enough to overcome their own fears. Ernie has turned into a very powerful healer."

On the subject of horseracing, James is adamant. "I'm currently rehabilitating two racehorses that were terribly damaged. I believe they were far too young to be racing. I would prefer that a horse not race until the age of five, but unfortunately, the industry won't make money that way. Because they're so young and they carry

JAMES FRENCH

all that weight on their back, they have back problems later on. One of them is named Shades, a beautiful horse but with a very nervous disposition. He won £86,000 in racing money, but as soon as he developed a back problem they turfed him out. That says it all for me. You can see he was born to run, there's no question about it—that horse was designed to run. But I can guarantee you he won his races because he was absolutely terrified. If you look at how a horse is ridden, it's got a bit in its mouth to stop, a stick to make it go faster, and a kick to make it go forward—all motivations based on fear. But there can be a whole different approach based on reward, and regard and trust.

"A few hundred people have trained with us and are now doing this work around the world. We've just begun the practitioner level for the Trust Technique. There are about twenty practitioners out there working at this level. I would say, with the animal communicators that we taught, and the Reiki healers that we taught, and now the Trust Technique practitioners, the work that we do has been amplified a hundredfold. And we have new practitioners starting out in the US, Canada, and different parts of Europe. I know if we keep teaching practitioners, we can put the Trust Technique out worldwide. Our message is all about relationship. It's also about regard, and about having peace of mind and sharing unconditional love with each other, not needy love, but unconditional love for a healing environment.

"I could turn every person I see into a healer for themselves and their animals."

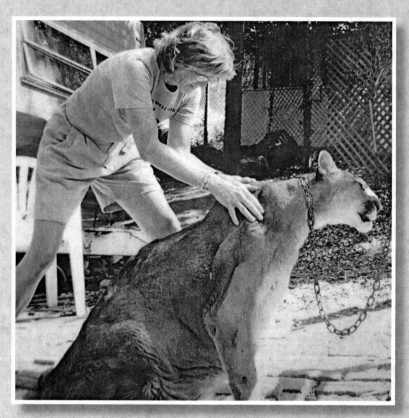

Dr. Haworth with Phoenix, the mountain lion at The Nature of Wildworks.
PHOTO: Dan Altchuler.

EILEEN HAWORTH

The Doolittles of Topanga Canyon

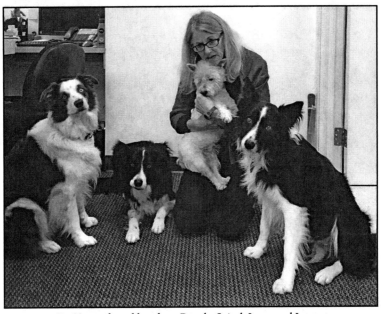

Dr. Haworth and her dogs, Dazzle, Spiral, Jessa, and Jargon.
PHOTO: Dan Altchuler.

Native-born Californian Eileen Haworth was newly married and fresh out of college with a degree in fine arts, and could not decide what she wanted to do. Her husband, Dan Altchuler, was about to set up a practice as a podiatrist. Thinking she might want to go into a related field, Eileen enrolled in the Los Angeles College of Chiropractic (later changed to the Southern California University of Health Sciences). Chiropractic interested her most, specifically sports medicine, and in 1979 she earned her degree of Doctor of Chiropractic.

Three years into her practice, in 1982, the National Olympic Committee called to ask if she would consider entering their selection process for people to work on the athletes—a first since there had never been a chiropractor on the Olympic team.

"I had been treating athletes with a now defunct club called Naturite Track Club. The coach of the club at that time had put more people on the U.S. Olympic Team than any other coach. When the Olympic Committee asked about a chiropractor, he gave them my name. I entered the selection process, ultimately for the Olympics, but basically it was to work at U.S. Olympic Committee-sponsored events. This Committee used to sponsor something called The National Sports Festival, a program to bring up young athletes and let them compete in international-style events. I was invited to work at a National Sports Festival in Indianapolis—I believe that was in 1982—and I spent a week or two in Indianapolis, working at that event. The following year, they asked me to another National Sports Festival in Colorado Springs. I stayed at the Air Force Academy for a couple weeks while they vetted me for the Olympic team."

Eileen Haworth became the first chiropractor to join the Olympic team's medical staff at the 1984 Summer Games in Los Angeles, and for the next seven years she continued to work with the Olympic Organizing Committee. Her life path seemed assured.

But then in 2002, Eileen received a tough cancer diagnosis. "At that time," she explains, "ovarian cancer had only a 10 percent survival rate. My prognosis was devastating: if I survived the first bout, I'd most likely have a second bout within three years, and most people do not survive that. It was the first time I ever thought, *Wow, I could be dead...* I was floored. It was the first time I had ever faced my own mortality. Suddenly, I knew I had to think about what I really wanted to do with my life. I had always been an animal lover and I always wanted to work with animals. It would be stupid to be lying on my deathbed and say 'Oh, damn, I didn't become an animal chiropractor.'"

This was her moment to put into practice—literally—her onetime dream of taking care of animals. "I decided I would do it now, but not partway. I would do it right."

First, she started treatments. She underwent surgery, chemo, and radiation, all the while making sure to stay well adjusted. She did Pilates exercise regularly, and had Reiki treatments.

Determined to be the best she possibly could, she enrolled in the Animal Veterinary Chiropractic Association course at the Parker College of Chiropractic, in Dallas, Texas. After graduation, she was certified by the Association and secured a position at the California Veterinary Hospital in Gardena, where she still works. One day a week she works at Northridge Animal Medical Center, in Northridge, California, and continues her practice as a chiropractor for humans in the office she shares with her husband.

"At first, very few veterinarians knew anything about chiropractic. When I thought I could be of help, I would try to talk them into letting me treat an animal. After all, they're educated one way and I'm educated slightly differently, so we had to find a way to come together. Now, more and more veterinarians are open to it and I've been able to work with them really well.

"One of the problems with veterinary medicine is that people often cannot afford to get the care their pets need. Charlie, a little Yorkie who couldn't walk, was brought to me, referred by a veterinarian who had seen him several times and had basically given up on him. He had done everything he could. X-rays didn't show the problem, because unless you have an eye for it, you don't always see subluxation—X-rays take pictures of bones; MRI's take pictures of soft tissue—and Charlie's owners couldn't afford an MRI. They had hit a dead end… The vet was about to suggest they put the dog down. But first he sent them to me.

"I examined the dog and found that he had an unlevel pelvis, which made walking so painful that he just stopped. I adjusted him and we made an appointment for the dog to come back the next week. The next week, I went into the waiting room and there he was. He was walking! It brought tears to my eyes.

"Veterinarians are basically internists; they are looking to save lives. Mechanical problems don't always cross their minds. The last time I saw Charlie was about six months ago; the owner comes back every so often to have the dog adjusted."

❧

On the subject of the soaring costs of veterinary care, Eileen agrees it's awful. "But," she argues, "running an office myself, I know how expensive it is. There are the people who have to be paid—a tech, someone to answer the phone—and then there's the equipment—X-ray machines, ultrasound machines, etc. So, when somebody is facing surgery that's going to cost $5,000, that's a lot of money. And it doesn't necessarily include follow-up visits or the care the animal has already received, or another MRI that might be needed. I don't know that much about insurance for animals. Some clients tell me that their insurance is fantastic, and others say it's really not worth it. Of course, some pet insurers pay for chiropractic.

"I have a West Highland White Terrier that I adopted. Her owners had come to our practice asking to have the dog put down because she kept peeing in the house. We were the fourth veterinary hospital they'd been to, initially searching for some sort of treatment, but each one told them the same thing, that the dog had become incontinent, just as humans sometimes do. The poor people were beside themselves. They had three kids and couldn't afford to keep going to veterinarians. I asked if they really wanted to put the dog down and they said no, but they couldn't afford the vet bills and they couldn't have her constantly peeing in the house. I knew some Westie rescue people, so the owners signed the dog over to me. The vet and I both agreed we would find the cause of the Westie's incontinence.

"Turns out she had a hip problem. The vet performed surgery on her and I did the rehab. Then I got in touch with the rescue people, but by then the dog was living with me and I couldn't let her go. Fourteen years later, I still have Jessa and no, she no longer pees in the house. She does have a leg-length difference in her back end, which throws her pelvis out of alignment. Jessa gets more manipulation than any other dog I own; she just stands there while I adjust her, and then she runs off and does her happy little dance.

"My friend, Mollie Hogan, owns a rescue facility for animals in the Santa Monica Mountains called The Nature of Wildworks, in Topanga, California. Mollie was once a lion tamer at the Los Angeles Zoo, but the Zoo got in trouble for its really bad conditions. They have since changed their ways, but back then they almost lost funding and were getting ready to lose their license. It was no fault of Mollie's, but she was let go and all the cats in her act were scattered. Finally, she managed to get them all back and launched The Nature of Wildworks.

"Mollie asked me to adjust one of her mountain lions, Phoenix, the only one that was really manageable. Up in years, he had arthritis and wasn't doing well. So periodically she had me come and adjust him. Phoenix loved it! They'd bring him out on a chain, walking him like a dog on a leash, and he'd sit or sometimes stand while I adjusted him, and he'd purr. Phoenix lived to around twenty or twenty-one.

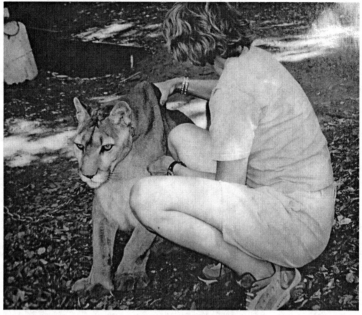

Dr. Haworth working on Phoenix, the mountain lion at The Nature of Wildworks. PHOTO: Dan Altchuler.

"My practice consists of a lot of dogs that do sports—like agility, conformation, and fly-ball—as well as nose work and tracking. I also treat arthritic dogs. They're brought to me to keep them in alignment, to stay in good health, increase range of motion, and decrease pain.

"The minute a patient comes in from the waiting room, I watch to see how it is moving. Dogs need to use almost every muscle, bone, and joint in their body to take a single step. They flex and extend from the top of the neck, C1, to the occiput (bump at the back of the skull). You can find the occiput by placing your finger behind your ear on the indentation; the bone above that is the occiput. Flexion also occurs at the base of the neck and at the lumbosacral junction near the tail. The thoracic spine rotates; it is located above the ribs. But because the function of flexion and extension is so important, the animal has to be able to flex and extend its neck and low back in order to move. So, I watch very closely as they walk. If I see anything unusual, I'll call it to the owner's attention. I may also watch the dog move toward and away from me, and making a big circle around me. Moving in a circle puts increased stress on the inside legs, which accentuates any lameness.

"I like to sit on the floor with the animal so that it has no fear of falling off a table. I ask the owner to get on the floor with us. And then, no matter what the problem may be, I start from the back and move forward, palpating as I go. My fingers tell me what I need to do as I move the joints. If I feel an area that isn't moving well, that's where I adjust. I let my fingers do the walking. I palpate each joint, not just the spine, but all major joints, even to the ribs.

"An adjustment can relieve pain that affects bones, joints, and even some organs, because of the pressure put on the nerves. Even the weight of a dime on a spinal nerve can cause pain."

Eileen has been entering her dogs in agility competitions for over sixteen years. "Because I'm biomechanically oriented, the importance of flexion and extension and full range of motion is of great interest to me—as is my interest in the biomechanics of movement. Which is part of what makes me a good chiropractor. Just as family veterinarians are trained to treat internal problems, my main thing is mechanics.

"One of my five dogs is a sixteen-year-old Border collie, a rescue who's an old gentleman and such a sweet little guy. They all work in my people office as therapy dogs. The Border collie just enters the room and lies down while I'm working. Most people are thrilled to have a dog sleeping in the room while they're being treated. My Westie is actually my best therapy dog because she is so portable. If my husband is injecting somebody or doing something that is painful, lots of people ask to have her in their lap."

Eileen and Dan make their home in Topanga Canyon, California, with their ménage of Border collies, Dazzle, Spiral, Jargon, Cache, and Jessa, their West Highland terrier, a Morgan horse named Topaz, and a miniature horse, Cooper.

"It's now been fourteen years and I never had that second bout of cancer that would have taken my life," Eileen says.

One can't help but wonder if her love of animals and that life-changing decision to heal them was what ultimately saved her life.

MARGRIT COATES

An Urgent Message

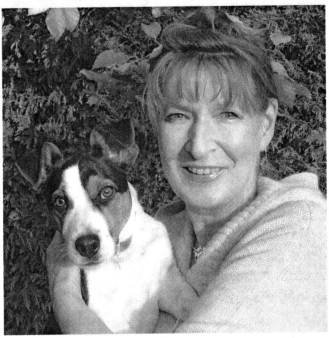

Margrit Coates, a leading animal healer and a renowned communicator. PHOTO: ©Margrit Coates.

Your best friend has something to tell you. To hear what that is, according to animal communicator and author Margrit Coates, you have only to tune in and listen.

"Our animal companions have wisdom they want to share with us; they possess great understanding that can help us along our paths. Each animal has a story—all animals: dogs, cats, birds, horses, dolphins, coyotes, wolves, bears. The human race is not the master species; it is the dominant species."

Speaking of her childhood in the north of England, Margrit remembers having always assumed that everybody was as sensitive and empathic as she was. She could easily sense when someone was troubled or unwell, and just by putting her hands on a person, he or she would immediately feel better. Young Margrit never thought about what she was doing; to her it was quite normal.

"The dogs and cats and horses I saw around me were actually communicating with me, mind-to-mind, soul-to-soul. I used to wonder why anyone would shout at a dog or a cat or behave in a nonempathic way—why didn't they understand them? Couldn't they hear them? Why did they not realize that animals are in their own world with their own language and their own feelings? And then it hit home: I was surrounded by humans who just weren't tuning in. Somewhere along the line, humans had fallen out of sync with animals."

Margrit's parents divorced when she was very young, and the family was poor. Entertainments for Margrit and her younger sister were few. "Without luxuries to distract me, I came to depend on nature and the surrounding wildlife, taking long walks and tuning in to whatever animals were around.

"I made my way through school and got a good education. After I earned my degree in art design, I started working in advertising in London. At the same time, I took workshops and clinics and courses in healing topics, and practiced Transcendental Meditation every day. I did that for ten years, which is why I now find it so easy to slip into the healing wavelengths. There can be a lot going on around me, but with the discipline of all those years of meditation, I'm able to shift consciousness into that state where I need to be to help the animals."

When the company Margrit was working for downsized in 1996, she lost her job. This undisguised blessing was the prompt she needed to exit the hectic business world and follow her heart's desire instead.

"I took one private college course, and another state college course in several areas of complementary medicine. When I was working with humans, I was able to help a woman who was terminally ill with cancer. She had become so much more peaceful and energized that she asked me if I could help her horse, who was not well. I did, and after that, other people started asking me if I would work with their animals.

"By this time, I was a registered healer and had my own clinic. I decided I needed to find out about animal healing. I discovered that the wavelength for healing and for interspecies communication is the same. I had always naturally combined the two because as we become healers, we're opening ourselves up to hear what animals say.

"My husband and I now live near the south coast of England, not far from the city of Southampton in a national park with thousands of free-roaming ponies. I have two grown stepchildren, and at the moment I have two cats. I often look after a friend's dogs, but I don't have dogs of my own because I travel so much. I don't have horses now for the same reason. I made a decision to make myself available to the world to offer clinics, lecture, and do TV interviews. The luxury of having a lot of animals would prevent me from being available for the teaching work.

"My mission, my purpose, and my passion is to help people better understand animals, to help them develop empathy and return to their healing nature. Every human has the ability to channel healing energy, to connect to the Source—whatever one thinks that Source is.

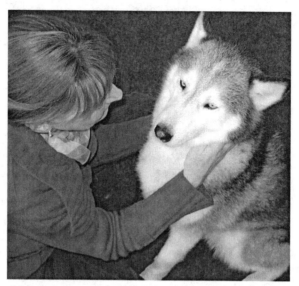

*Margrit Coates with her hands over the eighth major chakra,
found only in animals.* PHOTO: ©Margrit Coates.

"You know, we can go through life listening to one of two sources, either the clamoring of ego or the small still voice of soul. The ego seeks attention and material gain, power, and admiration. The soul seeks peace and understanding and the wisdom of other lifeforms, other sentient beings. We all have a choice: Do we want to dance to the ego, or do we want to go hand in hand with the soul?

"This is a time when animals urgently need to speak to us about climate change, because we are destroying their habitat, in the jungles, on the prairie, in the forest—everywhere. In destroying their habitat, we're of course destroying the human habitat too. We need our trees for oxygen and for the millions of species of rainforest herbs that could cure every disease on this planet. We are destroying everything we need, all of the medicinal blueprints and healing intelligence found within the plants. And the oxygen. When we cut down a forest, we change everything

—even the winds. And the winds will then change the course of rivers and seas and tides. So, we're destroying ourselves. That's what the animals, over and over again, are trying to get across in a big global message."

Margrit believes this is why the animals are beginning to speak up so clearly right now. They are trying to tell us that it doesn't have to be like this, "trying to bring us home," she says, "home to our true purpose. They are seeking peace just as humans are, and they are trying to lead us to the place where we'll find that peace. Our pets are our guardians, and our angels in animal form."

In her day-to-day work with animal companions, Margrit observes that more and more they are breaking through to speak out. And what she hears is: "Tell my person that I know everything about them. Tell them to please review the way they're living their lives—to look at their health, look at how they relate to others. Look at what they're eating, their lifestyle. If they spend their days playing with a cell phone, what space is there for spirituality?"

About circuses, Margrit is adamant. "There is no place in our human society in this millennium for locking animals up and depriving them of freedom to use them for our entertainment. Humans have plenty of ways to be entertained; we do not need to take away the freedom of wild animals. I worked with the last circus elephant in the UK who was rescued and is now in a place of sanctuary. It was harrowing for me to work with her. She was severely traumatized, taken from the wild as a three-year-old and beaten into submission, living her whole life—fifty-six years—in the circus. That elephant is a sentient being with thoughts and feelings! Humans need to get over thinking they're the only ones who have preferences and feelings. There are so many animals trying to communicate their pain, and humans are missing the messages.

"The healer isn't immune to the toxicity of our planet. Eleven years ago, I had a bout of breast cancer. That was a great learning curve, not only of suffering, but also of battling to regain my health. Three weeks after I was diagnosed I discovered a lump on my cat's chest. I immediately took her to the vet who performed a biopsy. 'I'm sorry to tell you,' he said, 'that this is a very rare form of mammary cancer in cats.' My cat was beyond help. 'Take her home,' he said. 'In two weeks' time, she will have deteriorated. Bring her back then.'

"I knew that she had been taking the energy of my cancer from me. I had dealt with my illness with complementary medicines, going to doctors who specialized in lots of different healing modalities. I did the same for my cat. She had acupuncture, she had homeopathy, and of course I was giving her constant healing.

"Two weeks later she was eating again, and she was lively. I took her back to the vet then and again another two weeks after that. This continued for a few weeks until one day the vet said, 'You don't need to keep bringing her in for check-ups. Just bring her back when she stops eating and you can tell it's the end.'"

But by now, kitty's body had other ideas. "Her tumor simply disappeared. They'd told me it was metastatic and highly aggressive, and that it had already metastasized. It was everywhere. It was the highest grade—all of the tests came back and confirmed it. And that was it. But now it was gone.

"When I scooped my cat up into my arms, I heard her say, 'Your cancer's gone now, too.' And I knew that it was. I just knew it had departed. She knew; her message was so strong.

MARGRIT COATES

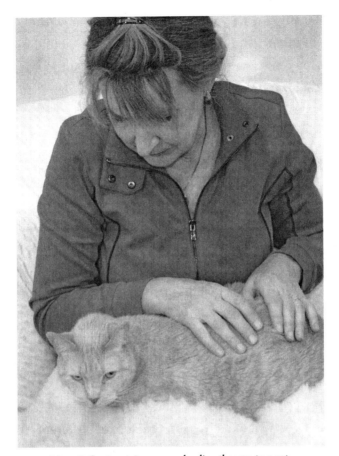

Margrit Coates giving energy healing therapy to a cat.
PHOTO: ©Margrit Coates.

"Well, four years went by and she was great. She lived until she was eighteen and died of old age. She did deteriorate some with age, and had become arthritic, but the cancer never returned.

"I too (knocking wood here) made a full recovery. Doctors signed off on me. So, she was my healer. I'm so humble about her. She's a far greater healer than I will ever be, because she was able to take my cancer from me. She guarded against the cancer taking my life.

"She's gone now and I miss her terribly. Not every relationship we have with every animal is going to be the same, or as deep.

All relationships with animals are unique; I know that each one will be different. And in that difference, I am actually evolving and moving on. I don't want to stand still. I want to learn from a whole host of animals. Who else is out there whom I can be sure to gain from and evolve through?"

Margrit has learned that all we are is a soul; all the rest is peripheral. What we achieve and become in life is all that we take with us. We cannot bring along any personal possessions. When her mother passed on, Margrit was struck by the fact that everything she had—her spectacles, her shoes, her purse—was just left there. All we own is our soul, and that is what we take with us. Everything else is a distraction. Of course, we need money for food and for fuel and the necessities of living. And we should be very careful on a day-to-day basis to shun involvement in destructive or even slightly inharmonious practices that leave a bad legacy. We also need to give back.

"One of the questions I often put to animals is, 'What is it about your people that made you choose them?' One animal said it was the light inside that person that looked different to her than everyone else's. It is magical; it is truly magical.

⁓❧

"My mission is to help people to hear their animal's message. It's through being present, through listening, that our pets' profound messages are heard. They are signposts to a great wisdom, great understanding. They all have a deep understanding of energy, the cosmos, each other, and of us, their beloved companions."

ANTHONY GEORGE

West Meets East

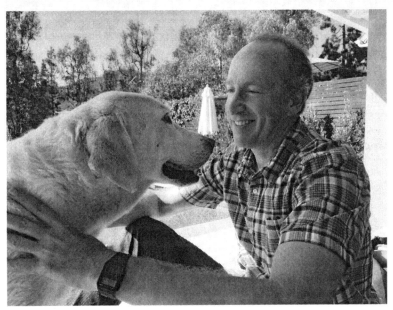

Lucky prefers her acupuncture treatments outdoors.

nthony George (Tony) DVM, knew from the age of nine that he wanted to be a veterinarian. At fourteen, he was able to get a work permit so he could work at the Pedro Point Animal Hospital in his hometown of Pacifica, California, cleaning the cages and taking the dogs out for walks along the cliffs by the ocean. His adoptive parents, high-school teacher father and homemaker mother, were able to put Tony through veterinary school by supplementing their incomes selling Amway out of their garage. He remembers the first family pet, a basset hound named Coco, and the shingled A-frame doghouse his father built and young Tony helped to paint. And how on cold and windy nights when the fog rolled in from the sea, he would crawl into the doghouse and curl up with Coco. "Ever since then, my dogs have always slept on my bed. I find it to be an almost caveman kind of thing, a communal connection."

He earned his BS in zoology and entered veterinary school at UC Davis; after graduation, he did his internship at a hospital in Hermosa Beach, California. From there he took a job at a small animal hospital in Santa Monica where he still is, twenty-five years later.

Early on, he began to hear about acupuncture from people who were having treatments done on their dogs and how much it was helping. "At that point all I had to offer was nonsteroidal anti-inflammatories, steroids, and muscle relaxants—and sometimes the medicine didn't work or it made the animals sick. I felt I was really hitting a wall. It was sad, because people adored their animals and I really wanted to help them. Acupuncture interested me. Around for at least 5,000 years, it's been used not only on people but on the animals that were important to them, like their horses, which they used for travel and warfare.

"I decided to learn more about acupuncture and got my certification from the International Veterinary Acupuncture Society. Many of the courses were taught by Doctors John Limehouse and his wife Priscilla Taylor Limehouse, trailblazers in the field of veterinary acupuncture and herbs. Eager to share their knowledge, after I passed the course they let me hang out with them and continue learning at their clinic in North Hollywood.

"In 1997, I started doing acupuncture and was one of the few veterinarians in Los Angeles who did. My very first patient was a little two-year-old terrier named Binky who had serious kidney disease. He wasn't eating well, he drank water nonstop, and urinated constantly, even on the bed. A full workup, including an ultrasound and kidney biopsy, showed congenital nephrosclerosis, meaning the kidney tissue was actually scarring.

"Binky's owner asked me if I thought acupuncture might help. I was totally new to it, but explained that I did at least know the acupuncture points for the kidney and for the appetite. I told her I would try. I wouldn't charge her, and we'd see what happens. So I gave the dog a treatment, just some basic acupuncture points, nothing fancy. The very next day, Binky's owner called me and said, 'Oh my God, he didn't pee all night. He didn't pee on the bed. He's eating better and he's not drinking a lot.'

"Okay... Great... I really wasn't expecting one treatment to do that much. She kept bringing Binky back once a week and he started to put on weight. I checked his kidney values; they had normalized. I was quite amazed as I am also a Western practitioner and I believe in science, and at the time, this was hard to comprehend. I almost felt as if the Fates had given me a gift. They were saying, 'Here you go. It's a gift! We'll give you some mess-ups down the road, but we're going to give you this one just so you know there's something to all this.'

"I continued to treat that dog; his kidney values continued to be normal and he lived to a ripe old age. It was well documented that he did indeed have that disease and I didn't do anything else to treat him. I just used acupuncture. It was my first acupuncture case and I was sold, I was a believer. I don't consider it alternative medicine—I consider it the original medicine."

Tony says he has a problem with being called a healer. "Because to me, it's not something that you say you are; it's something that, if you're fortunate, might be the result of what you do. People bring me their pets when much of the time, unfortunately, they have waited until things are really bad and it's a matter of too little too late. The animal is really deficient, or their disease is too far along and there's not a lot you can do; you might help just a little.

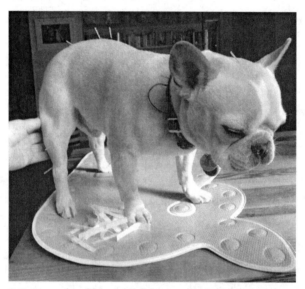

Frites is so relaxed he can hardly stay awake during his treatment.
PHOTO: A. Buffin.

"But then there're the 'wow' cases. One was a little Pekingese terrier with big round eyes and a pushed-in nose. His owners belonged to a Buddhist temple out in the Valley and they had driven two hours to see me. The dog was dragging both of his hind legs, which were not working at all. When you assess a dog, you look at the nerve function. You turn the foot under, and if they flip it back, that's great, because that's the first thing to go. Deep pain is the last thing to go. If you pinch a dog's toe, you want him to turn his head to see what you just did. If he doesn't, it means there is significant damage and the dog needs to get to a surgeon. When I pinched his toe he responded a little, but it really wasn't good."

Tony explains that IVDD (intervertebral disc disease) can be mild or it can involve a disc that has herniated into the spinal cord, causing compression and death of the spinal cord. There's a whole continuum of IVDD. The dog's owner told Tony that it had been going on for a month or more, which Tony felt made it even worse; if the condition is caught right away and the disc can be decompressed surgically, the pressure is removed and the spinal cord might regain function. When it's been going on for a long time, the prognosis is not as good. Tony told the dog's owner he needed to take the dog to a surgeon. Right away. *Today.*

"A great believer in Traditional Chinese Medicine (TCM), the man pleaded with me to treat his dog with acupuncture, reminding me that he had driven two hours to see me. Finally I agreed, on the condition that he would go see a surgeon. Then I put the needles into the dog—again, basic points, points around where I thought the lesion was, and distal points, meaning points away from the problem area on the head side and the tail side. It was one of my evening appointments and they left right after the treatment.

"The next day I called to make sure he went to see a surgeon.

"'He's walking,' the owner said.

"'That can't be right.'

"'Yes, he's walking.'

"'No, that just can't be right!'

"I thought maybe the dog was dragging his leg and he mistook that for walking. But the following week when he brought him in, the dog was actually walking! He walked like a drunken sailor, but he was definitely walking. And he was no longer incontinent. That was the other really big miracle. It was truly amazing.

"One thing I know about medicine: In the movies, someone will say, 'The doctor told me I have one week to live.' Nobody knows that! Nobody knows how much time you have. There're so many variables and so many factors that can affect healing: the degree of trauma or damage or the extent of the disease, and one's own inherent constitution. We've all seen people who are bulletproof: they keep falling down only to get right back up. And then there are people who just can't catch a break. They get pneumonia, they get this cancer and that cancer. In Traditional Chinese Medicine it's called your prenatal jing, which is basically what you were given. It's your allotment.

"That's what I really like about Chinese medicine. It makes so much sense. I'm not against Western medicine. I love Western medicine, I practice Western medicine. If you have pneumonia, I don't have a problem with antibiotics. If you have a broken leg, we can usually fix it, fix it surgically, and then use Traditional Chinese Medicine to balance things out later on. In Western medicine, if you have high blood pressure—here, take a pill. You've got arthritis—take a pill. Whereas Chinese medicine asks, what are you eating? What's your diet? What kind of exercise do you do?

"Eastern medicine also wants to know your family history, your prenatal jing. What were you allotted? If you were dealt a bad hand of cards, you have to deal with that. But there are things you can do peripherally as far as diet, exercise, and your environment are concerned to enhance what you were given. On the flip side, you may have been dealt some great cards, but then mess up your game by eating bad food, drinking too much, or smoking."

Tony identifies stressors in just about every aspect of modern life. "We're cortisol-driven. People are stressed out, struggling to make ends meet, dealing with family problems, personal problems, world problems, the planet, the environment. And all of that takes its toll. Cortisol causes a lot of problems. You see it every day in people's puffy faces and swollen ankles."

He describes how Chinese medicine is specific to each organism. "For instance, they'll look at your tongue, which is a bunch of blood vessels, a window into your vascular circulation. Is it pale? Is it red? Is there a yellow or white coating? Is it cracked? And they feel your pulses. Are they strong? Are they weak? Are they thready? It's a really simple way to look at someone's constitution.

"It may sound crazy at first, but once you learn about it, TCM makes sense. For instance, a spleen chi deficiency can lead to dampness in the lungs. In Chinese medicine, the spleen is the equivalent of the pancreas and is involved in digestion. The spleen/pancreas and lungs aren't typically associated with one another in Western medicine. That made sense to me the day I ate fast food at a drive-in and started to connect the dots. Afterwards, I felt like I couldn't breathe. Then I thought, *Oh, wait a minute. I'm eating this food, this processed food that's full of chemicals, and I'm having a reaction to it. I'm probably getting a release of histamine which causes fogginess and inflammation of the lungs.* And it all started coming together for me. When I do eat right, when I eat food that's not 'damp' for my constitution, I feel so much better. I can breathe better. I have more energy and I'm happier.

"I learned which foods are warming and which are cooling. But it gets even more complicated. What time of the year is it? If it's wintertime, maybe eat more warming foods. Eat stews. Eat root vegetables. Summertime? Have some watermelon. Have raw salad with some cucumbers.

"The same is true for our animals. I get clients who tell me they don't give their dogs any human food. Well, what's human food? Human food is high-quality dog food. There's not a dog chicken and a human chicken; there's chicken. Is it good chicken or chicken that's been discarded that they put into the dog food? You know, I understand that people are busy, and I'm not saying all dry dog food is bad. But if you think about it, would you want to eat the same dried thing every day for the rest of your life?

"We also see many diets that are inflammatory. If you eat something you are allergic to, you'll have an inflammatory reaction that seeps out into the joints, the lungs, the kidneys. And over time, it can cause chronic ailments. So I get really excited when I hear somebody talk about feeding pets fresh vegetables and fresh meats."

Tony feels that as with people, diet and exercise are important to an animal's health. In Chinese medicine, most disease processes are thought to be due to stagnation in the flow of chi. Needles are used to keep the chi flowing, as are exercise and a good diet.

Acupuncture has helped him put the pieces together. "I see animals that are born responders. If an animal is a really good responder, it really reacts to the needles. It's like anything else. Not every patient responds for every ailment every time. Just as in Western medicine, somebody can take one medicine, like an anti-inflammatory, and say, 'My God! The pain's gone. I feel so much better!' Somebody else can take the same medicine and get sick from it.

"After I'd been doing acupuncture in the clinic for about seven years, one day a woman came in with a cute little white Persian cat named Gia who was suffering from congestive heart failure. When she first came to the office, the cat got so freaked out from the dogs and the noise that her flesh turned blue. The woman was worried that Gia was going to have a heart attack right there in the hospital."

ANTHONY GEORGE

It occurred to Gia's human that since she lived just two blocks from the hospital, perhaps the doctor would consider coming to her house to treat Gia. This patient was the first of many in Tony's house-call practice.

From there it snowballed; Tony makes house calls regularly now, four days a week. He discovered that being treated in their home environment is always more relaxed for the animal, especially those that are especially anxious. Once the needles are in place, endorphins and serotonin are released, along with anti-inflammatory modulators.

One of Tony's calls was to a private rescue organization, "Friends of Animals," run by Martha Wyss, a woman in her eighties who became an inspiration to Tony. "Martha would take in dogs that nobody else wanted, always without judgement. Maybe the people were moving away, or had lost their job; for whatever reason, they had to give up their animals. Martha would provide food, shelter, and medical care, all the while trying to find her rescues a loving home. And if there was ever any problem, she'd take the animal back, no questions asked. People would drop off boxes of kittens, and if it was before weaning age, they'd have to be bottle-fed every couple of hours. It was really labor-intensive."

Tony remembers one dog, DJ, who had been adopted out and was brought back a few years later, his hind end paralyzed. The owner said the dog had fallen into a hole in the backyard. "DJ wasn't the friendliest of dogs; in fact, he would try to bite. I would go there and do acupuncture on him, but he remained paralyzed —another example of how it doesn't work for everything. I think he liked the attention, though. Both of the dogs I have now are from Friends of Animals.

"I try to push people toward adopting. There are a lot of other places that offer purebreds for adoption, like Lab Rescue, but when you have an animal that has a bunch of different breeds in him, you tend to get a healthier dog because they possess what's called hybrid vigor, the best components from each. I'm not saying anything against a purebred dog. But I just think of all the wonderful dogs that are already here and need a home.

"Being a vet can be extremely stressful. People bring you their cherished pets, animals that are really members of their family, and look to you to make recommendations on treatment and surgery, if necessary. There are of course times when your recommendations don't turn out the way you would have liked them to. It's heartbreaking when you have to look someone in the eye who has entrusted their loved one to you and tell them it's not going well. It's really, really horrible.

"That's where Traditional Chinese Medicine has taught me so much. That it's all about yin and yang: dark and light, female and male, cold and hot, peace and war, good and bad. There's always going to be good, but it's not *always* going to be good. And there's going to be bad, but it's not *always* going to be bad. It goes back and forth. Understanding that has really helped me.

"I also learned about the Five Elements, categories of constitutions in both people and animals. Certain animals or people may have a primary constitution, which can be a major consideration in their treatment. For instance, the liver is associated with wood. A terrier breed might be considered a "wood" breed—tenacious, take no prisoners and fight to the end; whereas the element of earth might be more in evidence in a Labrador—happy-go-lucky, loves everybody. But within those categories you can have a Lab that maybe has an edge, or you can have, say, a terrier that's really warm and loving. While not writ in stone, those are guidelines as to how to treat any given animal with acupuncture. Looking at the animal and its history, as well as figuring out what its element is, help in working out a treatment plan.

"The Five Elements has also been used to explain the Circle of Life, with each element folding into the next in a circle. Imagine the cycle starting with wood, as a plant that's growing, a time of growth and development. Then fire, which is like the teenage years—vibrant, emotional, erratic. The next element is earth, a time to settle down and raise a family. Then there is metal, a time to sit back and reflect on one's life. And finally, there is water, the kidney phase, a period of calm, toward the end of life. Then imagine the cycle beginning all over again: a pond of water with new shoots springing back up and new life coming through... the return to the wood element as the cycle continues. For me, that put a lot of the puzzle pieces together."

Tony expresses his passion beautifully. "I love animals and I love most people. To make something better—to have a hand in making something better—is my life. I can't think of many things that surpass that feeling."

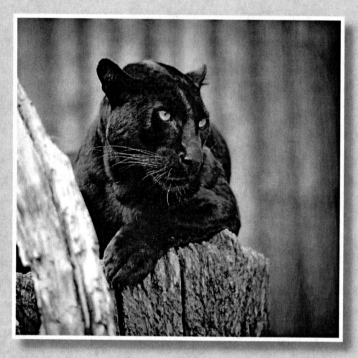

In a communication with Anna, a black leopard expressed that he did not like his name, Diablo, and was then renamed Spirit by his guardian, Jurg Olsen.

ANNA BREYTENBACH

A Walk in Anna's World

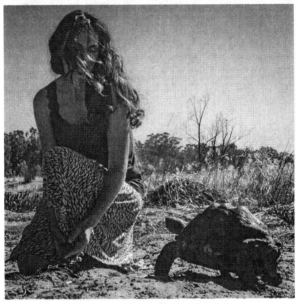

Anna Breytenbach with a wild tortoise.
PHOTO: James Kydd.

She stands silently, patiently, at the fenced-in night shelter at the Jukani Predator Park in South Africa, waiting for the black leopard named Diablo to show himself. With Anna is Jurg Olsen the manager of the sanctuary for big cats and his wife Karen. An ex-policeman turned conservationist, Jurg plays with and snuggles some of the other big cats in the park, but now he is at a loss. Diablo, a recent rescue from a European zoo, has been impossible to approach even on the opposite side of a fence. "This is a very dangerous animal," Jurg explains. "He looks at everyone as though he hates them and wants to kill them." Jurg was desperate, he didn't want to lose Diablo. As a last resort he agreed to invite world renowned professional animal communicator Anna Breytenbach to see if she can help.

"He won't let anyone near his shelter without snarling and baring his teeth," he warns. "The one encounter I had with him put me in the hospital for a week."

Just then the black cat emerges from the shadows and Jurg expects his usual angry greeting, but the moment Diablo sees Anna he becomes suddenly calm. He allows her to move closer to the fence where she kneels, not necessarily looking at him, just there in her utter stillness. Diablo relaxes, blinks his eyes. Several minutes go by, then Anna turns to Jurg. "This cat was badly abused at the zoo he was kept in. He's also very worried about the two young leopard cubs that were next to him at the zoo. And," she adds, "he doesn't like his name."

She goes on to relate details about Diablo's former life in the zoo that only the animal could have shared, all of which are subsequently confirmed. Jurg is stunned.

When Anna returns later that day to check on Diablo, the cat tells her that was the first time anyone related to him for who he was and he thanks Jurg for that. Jurg had thanked Diablo, too, for communicating with Anna. She laughs. "Then they thanked each other for the thanks."

Over the coming days, the cat's transformation brings tears to Jurg's eyes. For the first time in months, Diablo walks out of his shelter into the larger enclosure and sits contentedly on top of a tree stump. With a swish of his tail, he greets Jurg with a series of low grunts. Feeling somewhat foolish and self-conscious, Jurg tells Diablo that he is beautiful and would in the future be known as Spirit—the spirit of the sanctuary. "I now respect Spirit for what he is and how he wants to be treated."

❧

It seems wherever Anna goes, her quiet presence affects all wildlife: fish gather at her side when she swims; wild birds land on her shoulders; in primate territory, when she lies down in a field, a baboon comes and lies beside her and begins to groom her.

I sense evidence of that quiet presence when I interview her at her home in South Africa via Skype. Speaking softly in a lightly accented voice, Anna explains that animal communication is not a gift... "It's a simple matter of quieting the mind and intending to connect. The animals pick up on that right away, easily. I send either a mental image, a thought or an emotion, whichever comes most naturally at that moment and I receive messages back of remarkable clarity. I would define the term as a direct mind-to-mind communication or a transference of information, although it's as much a matter of the heart as the mind. We all have these abilities, they're hard-wired into the very design of our being. To our native ancestors, these skills were a part of everyday life; the trick is knowing how to access it intentionally instead of waiting for it to happen."

Born and raised in Cape Town, South Africa, Anna describes her upbringing as ordinary suburban with no special exposure to animals. "Although as a child I did have an over-developed sense of empathy with the non-human world. Even in junior school, I was always finding a way to make my homework assignments about one of the big cat species. Mind you, South Africa is a very civilized country—we don't have lions running in the streets. Most South Africans never get to see a lion or a leopard in their entire lives unless they can afford to go on safari. So, I don't know where that fascination of mine with big cats came from. Something from another realm calling to me, perhaps...."

Anna studied Psychology, Marketing and Economics at the University of Cape Town, and volunteered on weekends at a conservation education project where she also received training as a cheetah handler. After graduation, she entered the corporate world and for twelve years had a successful career in Human Resources and Information Technology which eventually took her to Australia and the US.

"I worked for a tech firm in downtown Seattle, and was able to indulge my love of nature by joining a hiking club on weekends. Eventually, I found that the hiking club folks were only interested in discussing the woes of the work week, so I joined the tracking club instead. A whole new mysterious world unfolded to me. Knowing nothing about North American animal species, I was following footprints that were totally strange to me. I would go to the tracking instructor out on the sand banks of the river or to the wolf-tracking instructor and describe excitedly in great detail a footprint I'd just seen and ask, "What animal is it?" To my frustration, I would not get an answer. Or the answer would be another question, one that would push me beyond my current knowledge and challenge me to look deeper. So I had to learn directly from coyote what coyote is.

"Where I was living, on a small island off the coast of Seattle, there was a wolf sanctuary. I volunteered there as a hands-on assistant, doing everything from scooping up wolf poop to writing fund-raising newsletters and education program material."

We talked about how strong her pull was to the natural world and her fascination with animals in the wild, and wondered if perhaps there was something way back in her ancestry.

She laughed. "Interesting that you mention that. I only recently discovered that the Breytenbach name, which is of German origin, has a family coat of arms with not only a wolf in it but all the instruments of torture and wolf trapping devices as well. Seems I come from a long lineage of wolf trappers! So I guess there is something in my heritage between humans and wolves, but obviously not pleasant. Maybe I'm making up now for what some of my ancestors did.

"I was working a fourteen-hour day Monday through Friday and devoting my weekends to following my passions. After a while, my weekends began to speak to me more loudly than my weekdays and I ended up having very little to say to my colleagues that wasn't about work. While on weekends, I was being drawn into states that were more about *being* rather than *doing*. That opened up quite a chasm between my weekday persona and my weekend self. I began to feel like a stranger in my own life and career.

"The kinds of projects I was working on in the corporate world were specifically aimed at making businesses more effective, which in some cases meant environmental pollution or destruction. If the gap hadn't been so uncomfortable, I might have taken even longer to leave."

"At one time I wanted to become a vet, but my family couldn't afford medical school. Now, looking back, I realize that volunteering at these various animal shelters and conservation programs over the years had in fact created an alternate resume for me. Not the formal qualifications I would have had if I had gone to veterinary school, but skills that were much closer to my heart. Those two years in Seattle spending weekends tracking or going on a bird language course or snowshoeing in the trail of mountain lion tracks, or even speaking to a bunch of drug-abusing

139

teenagers about wolf conservation, all had a more profound and lasting effect on me.

"I'm glad now that I didn't go the medical route because that version of science is separatist and it objectifies animals, whereas I come into the field sideways, from the angle of wellbeing and health. Because I am able to hear directly from the animals what is going on for them, I am able to shortcut the need for investigation. I cannot make a medical interpretation, a medical professional needs to do that, however I can simply relay the felt sensations on the part of the animal which can be helpful for a medical diagnosis."

I asked her to talk about her first inklings of her abilities. Most of the other healers I had interviewed described healing or telepathic experiences that began in early childhood and continued to develop over the years.

"It wasn't until I was thirty—rather late to come to telepathic communication—that I began to be consciously aware I was receiving information that could not otherwise be explained and subsequently discovering the information proved accurate. Yet, there were times I wondered if I was hallucinating, or if maybe I had some mental illness… or whether in fact something explainable was actually happening. Those questions prompted me to begin an online search where I discovered the whole field of telepathic communication. As I delved deeper, I found further explanations that accurately described my experiences.

"Even so, my analytical mind still found a host of reasons to explain it all away. For at least two years I was my own biggest skeptic—even after these incidents were being proved. It was amazing, the gymnastics my mind would go through. 'Oh, that was just a lucky guess, or perhaps I had subconsciously heard something earlier in the day'… my ego based mind kept trying to talk myself out of the fact that something larger was actually informing me. I decided then to take advanced level courses during my vacation days at the Assisi International Animal Institute where I met my mentor, Dr. Jeri Ryan, a beautiful, wise elder and psychologist. She kept gently encouraging me. She also designed exercises and programs that specifically allowed for validation and corroboration of data, which did a lot to appease my thinking mind. My other mentor was Jon Young who has studied indigenous cultures around the world and their profound connection to nature. The youngsters in those cultures grow up to be deeply related to the non-human worlds. If it were not for my two mentors, I might not be doing this today. With all that was going on inside of myself and feeling the increasing pressure that what I was doing was not really acceptable to the mainstream, I might have given up."

The subject of healing came up. I was curious to know if her communication with animals ever resulted in an actual healing. She remembered the incident with a cheetah she was working with in a captive cheetah program. "We used to run the cheetahs once a week for exercise. He was fine walking, but one day while running he wasn't able to take the turns. He was either completely overshooting the turns or not making them as tightly as before. As a result we had to run him less often because he'd also started to go off-track, which could be particularly dangerous to the humans who were managing him.

"One day, I was sitting quietly with the cheetah with my hand resting lightly on its shoulder and had the thought, 'Oh, how wonderful it must be to have a cheetah's body... if only I were that athletic....' I guess that imagined wish changed into an intention that was heard, because suddenly I felt my own body shape-change almost as if I were morphing into a cheetah's shape.

I then experienced an extension of my body going out beyond the end of my coccyx, as if I had a tail. I could even feel it swishing. About one-third along the tail's length I felt a very sharp burning pain and thought, *what's that?* Immediately, that thought popped me out of the experience of being in the cheetah's body. Back in my human body and fully wide awake, I ran my fingers down the length of the cheetah's tail and felt a little lump. I reported that to the managers of the facility.

"An X-ray showed a broken vertebra in the tail. Cheetahs use their tails as rudders when they are running, and when they turn, they whip their tail around; it's what steers them. With a broken vertebra he was unable to make the turns and could easily have injured himself."

I asked her if that experience prompted her to experiment further with healing.

Anna said it did. That sometimes when a friend's or a family member's pet was at the vet and the doctor seemed uncertain, Anna would tune in with the animal and ask one question: Show me your body on mine. Then, she explained, her body would become a map for the animal's. "So if the animal has an issue with his front left paw, I would experience it on my left hand. Other vets heard about me and would ask surreptitiously if I would check in with some of their animal patients."

She described one case of a dog that was refusing food and vomiting and wasn't responding to the meds. Yet his blood tests were normal. "So I asked the dog. I got an image from his perspective of himself with a fatty kind of food in front of him and not being able to tolerate it. Then I got an image of the fat being inside his stomach and his body rejecting it. I described exactly that to the vet. The vet said it sounded like it might be a pancreas problem because pancreatic enzymes are responsible for digesting fat. He tested for pancreatic enzymes and the dog was found to have pancreatic cancer.

"So you see how direct input from the animals can be very helpful to vets because the animals can tell me from their perspective what is or is not working for them. The anatomical and chemical explanation can come later. With the use of telepathic communication the animals can let us know what they're experiencing, which can help in the healing.

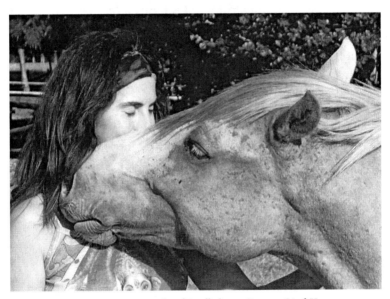

Anna communicating with a friendly horse. PHOTO: Liesl Kruger.

"There are other kinds of healings," Anna explains. "There is the emotional healing that comes about when the animal feels seen and heard, and knows that his truth is being acknowledged with compassion by another being. When we tune in, we are essentially syncing into resonance with the animal so that we are literally on the same wave length, the same frequency. When we humans can make ourselves present, to be in the here and now—which is where all non-humans reside—then we are in sync with them. And by the way, that goes two ways, sending and receiving; it is a two-way knowing of each other. I'm not doing a disembodied psychic reading on an animal, or using imagery or psychometry or a crystal ball or a pendulum; it's a direct connection with the animal's essence; they are fully knowing and seeing me in that moment as well.

"Horses read us particularly well. They are very good at reflecting to humans what they are really feeling; it is for us to know them. So even before communication, there's just connecting in that beautiful space of openness."

That led Anna onto the subject of our own healing. "The same applies if we can turn from *inter-species* to *intra-being*. I've used this myself when I've been ill—I had a number of serious illnesses, like malaria. I've had some amazing miraculous healings of my own body without chemical intervention or any other drastic measures by reaching a kind of agreement with the various organisms that are living inside my body. We humans are largely bacteria that are fully sentient in their own way. So the matter of healing for me is always about the deeper impulses and causes than just what appears to be manifesting physically. When we communicate within our own bodies or with any other being that is in distress, and we can find the reasons behind the physical distress, then we can find out what is needed at those mental, emotional, spiritual levels to bring about a physical healing.

On the subject of meditation, I was curious to know if that was something she practiced daily or did she just slip into it when the moment requires it. "Apparently, this is what I hear from people who watch me. I don't know that of myself because it has become so second nature. And don't get me wrong, I am fully in my humanness, my persona, and I get triggered as much as anyone. I have my bad days, and my reactions to things. But when there is a need or a situation in the moment, whether it's a pigeon lying injured on the road in front of the car on a busy highway or a lion in the wilds of Africa, people who happen to be around me see my state of being change: they describe me as still, serene, very present, and very grounded. I think staying grounded is important. It's not about ascending to some mysterious other realm or having to float off on some mantra to activate my twenty-second strand of DNA. Nothing could be more natural and grounded than sinking into the present moment. I don't do it deliberately any more. When there's a spontaneous need from whatever is calling me in the environment, I get to that state quickly and naturally. I'm not aware of it myself, because I am not orchestrating it.

"It's almost as if I experience myself as pure energy; I'm just in the flow, and everything else is flowing around me at that moment, there's no resistance. It's a very lovely state to be in, and I have to say that one needn't attend workshops for telepathic communication to access these states. Other practices in my life have really helped me get there much more quickly, and help with my clarity in telepathic communication. Like a very casual yoga practice, nothing particularly devoted or consistent, and breathing practices, stillness, meditation—any personal practice that gets me out of my thinking mind. I align myself with my own animal body which makes the animal kingdom more accessible to me."

I wondered if it is something of a balancing act for her in her work and her everyday life. Was there some sort of line between her work and doing the laundry or having lunch with friends? How does that work?

She laughed. "That's a very good question. And the answer to that is both yes and no. I have to keep up with all of the usual in my life, running a home and organizing the logistics of traveling around the world giving workshops and lectures. Part of the problem in the balancing act is that my mind is quite strongly analytical and that sometimes keeps me from paying attention to my intuition.

"By the same token, it's fun to play with in daily life when I do. I can have lost my way, and the phone batteries are dead and there's no navigation or GPS available, and I have no written directions. Then it's, oh well, let's just feel which way to go. And seven turns later, there I am, on some obscure street, right at the meeting I'm meant to be at, using intuition alone.

"I also use my intuition about what food is good for me. Because whatever you read, you'll find arguments on either side of the case for some particular food or eating protocol. Instead of paying attention to any concepts or the most recent research, I feel an internal *yes* or *no* or *not now* for what I'm thinking about eating or drinking; I feel drawn to one food or another. As a result, I do have a very healthy diet based on what is right for this body at this time."

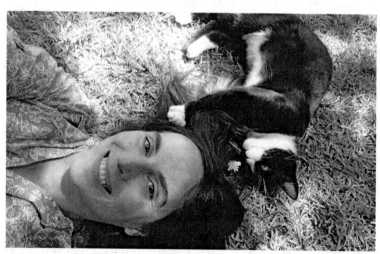

Anna with one of her kitties. PHOTO: Anna Breytenbach.

ANNA BREYTENBACH

Asked about what pets Anna has at her house and how she communicates with them, she says, "I'm lucky enough to live with three kitty companions, and the telepathy is flowing all the time. Animals are not inclined to make small talk, so I don't use telepathy for the sake of it. But I live on the edge of a forest, and there are lynx and leopard around, so my cats need to be in before dark or else they might not survive the night. They have an indoor-outdoor lifestyle, they can come and go as they please because I had already telepathically communicated with them and explained the dangers. I didn't have to use any restraining method; instead I created a picture of a cat much bigger than they are chomping down on them, and them having a very painful death. I got their very attentive agreements to come in to avoid that fate. That was a one-time conversation about two years ago. Now, all I do when it's getting close to sunset and they're out somewhere off on their own adventures, is I simply send a little heart connection, a little heart greeting to them that it's time to come in. Then from their perspective I imagine looking back at the house, the view of the house emerging larger and larger into their fields of vision. I do that with each of them in turn. It's never been longer than five minutes before they come back. I have not used my voice. I have not called them. I haven't shaken the kitty treat bag. Because two years ago, my cats each agreed to this and they are kind enough to honor their agreement.

"Oh yes, it works with all animals. But don't forget, it is always the animal's choice. They are sentient beings, self-aware, and they always make their own choices. So, if it doesn't bring results, it may just be that they have heard us loud and clear but they choose to be off on their adventure following some delicious trail.

"People can use telepathy with obedience training, too. It's kind of a fun way to teach them. I've had people in my workshops prove it to themselves. Instead of giving the instructions verbally like stay or heel, I encourage them to try it silently, telepathically. And it works.

"Because for young animals having to learn how to be successful in the human world is quite a thing. Every household has its different rules, different routines, different energies. We can use telepathy to explain to them both our feelings and our wishes in mental images showing them why we want them to do something. For instance, when you take the puppy outside, actually imagine the feeling of having to urinate. And send a mental image to the dog of crouching down or lifting the leg. They get the memo, they really do.

"So much of dog training is based on dominating the animal. How often do we hear, 'You've got to let them know you're the pack leader?' Well, the dogs are not stupid, they know we're not dogs. They don't expect us to be leaders. They will look to us for guidance and for decisions. But so many domination-based training methods are based on fear. It amazes me how often people who are well-intentioned animal lovers actually end up using fear as a way to control and manage the animal. And they think it works. 'Look. The animal is obeying me now.' No, that animal is just trying to avoid the pain of punishment. But it's a dead relationship, you've got an animal that is resentful and certainly feeling quite helpless. It's disempowering and dishonoring; a very unfulfilling relationship all around."

We got on the subject of the health of the planet. I was curious to know her thoughts. I asked her if she thinks it's too late to change this destructive course we're on. In one of the interviews I saw, Anna talked about the eleventh hour, fifty-ninth minute. How do we change that?

"Changing the planet is really about reconnecting with the planet. And I personally know of no better way to do that than

ANNA BREYTENBACH

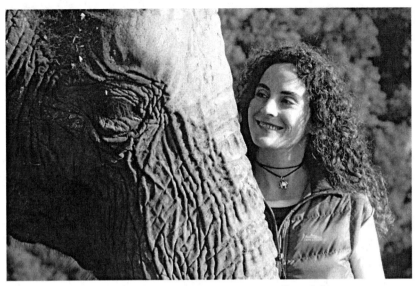

Anna with Ellie the elephant. PHOTO: Geoff Daiglish.

to re-establish relationships with non-humans in everyday life. It can be with the earth while mowing your lawn. It can be with the bird that flies overhead. Sending out a little acknowledgement that you've seen them, and you appreciate their song, or their beauty, or their purpose. You know, if we can appreciate a song bird with the same non-judgmental gratitude as we can a cockroach in our kitchen, then we're getting somewhere. Then we are changing the world, not because we are attached to the outcome, but because we ourselves are being in the frequency that is healing, and that is uplifting."

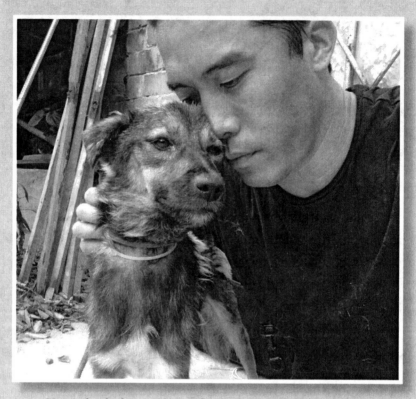

Marc with a dog he carried out and rescued with 1000 other dogs from a slaughterhouse at the Yulin Dog Meat Festival.

MARC CHING

Undercover Angel

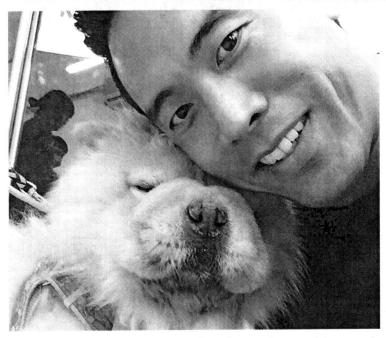

Marc Ching with Lion, who was shot with a pellet gun, electrocuted, beaten and burned. She was rescued on his first trip to China, and now lives in Massachusetts.

UP TO NOW, we have been in the company of angels of every stripe possessing all sorts of skills and performing them on all sorts of species—two-legged, four-legged and winged. Like all angels, they are selfless and dedicated and determined to improve the lives of every sentient being that comes their way.

Having brought these angels to the pages I thought my work was done. Until I happened upon one more healer who works quietly in the corner of a small store in a suburb of Los Angeles. His calm and focused demeanor as he listened to a pet owner, at the same time zeroing in on the pet at the person's side, intrigued me. I had to know more.

Little did I suspect that in learning more about him, I would be following him into an unexpectedly dark place, a place of evil I never knew existed. A place that reminds us of the tenuous fault line between good and evil, angels and demons, that runs through the landscape of humanity. The temptation to avert one's eyes is great. Yet, the force of Marc's bravery—and yes, heroism, would not let me look away. *Warning: this story of Marc Ching marked me.*

⁓✿

On a busy street in the suburbs of Los Angeles is a small, unassuming store with the odd name, Petstaurant. Street parking is iffy; you might try around back where there are two designated spots. Once inside, you weave your way past stacks of cartons containing frozen containers of food, supplements, bags of bones and snacks. Then you step around the several dogs milling around, some belonging to customers; others, it turns out, are Marc Ching's rescues.

At first, it seems a ragtag operation, but then the eyes wander to the far corner of the store where Marc sits at a wooden table in deep consultation with a woman, a golden retriever at her feet. Marc strokes the dog, examines the eyes and teeth, then rubs the inside of the dog's ears, leaning down to sniff them. He makes notes on a yellow pad. "Yeast dermatitis," he says, and lays out a diet protocol of freshly cooked meat and vegetables that can be cooked at home or bought at the store, along with supplements.

The woman standing next to me tells me that her dog had the same condition; her vet had been trying to get rid of the condition for months with no success, after which Marc had cleared it up in two weeks. A man with a Labrador mix tells me he's here for a follow-up; his dog had inflammatory bowel disease which Marc also cured in a matter of weeks.

Marc does not charge for these consultations and healing sessions, only for the food and supplements he prescribes. The food is all organic, freshly cooked every day at a kitchen across town. Free of artificial and processed ingredients, grains or starches, which he believes can exacerbate certain health problems, the menu includes a wide variety of meats, poultry, fish, vegetables, and herbs.

After his last appointment, he goes to his other office a few miles away where he conducts human healing sessions for which he does charge. "You can put dogs on a protocol and they'll get better quickly; people, though, can go out and do drugs and drink alcohol and not stick to the protocol, which makes the healing more complicated and can take longer."

Marc is Hawaiian-born, thirty-seven years old, slim and fit, with short black hair and dark, serious eyes. He is married to Linda, who is of Chinese descent. They have two children, Brendon, five, and three-and-a-half-year-old Kyrsten. The adopted son of a well-to-do family, Marc chose not to join the family business—his father, two brothers, and sister are all stockbrokers. Instead, he left home at seventeen to go to the mainland. At that point, he faced a severe identity crisis; bearing the emotional scars of a child given up for adoption by a teenage mother, he had never fully dealt with his feelings about this until his own teenage years. Then he began getting into trouble and using drugs. Until the day when Marc suddenly saw that he had to seriously rethink his life. For that, he turned to the animals, remembering the love he always had for them, and they for him, as a child.

Growing up, his greatest teacher was his grandmother, a fifth-generation herbalist and expert in Traditional Japanese Medicine. Marc found himself giving more and more thought to his grandmother's teachings about healing and nutrition. He decided to further his education and earned a bachelor's and then a master's degree in business administration, finally returning to the study of holistic medicine. Mila, the small pit bull mix that Marc had in college, developed a fatal inflammatory bowel disease that his vet was unable to treat. Realizing that given the proper food and supplements his dog might have been healed, Marc was moved to delve more deeply into the practice of holistic medicine, both for animals and humans. Following the teachings of his grandmother, who firmly believed that the cause of any ailment usually has to do with poor nutrition, Marc began to experiment. The result was starch and grain-free pet food, samples of which he took to farmers markets.

A year later, using every credit card he could get his hands on, he opened his first business, Petstaurant, a storefront for his line of food that also included a shelter and his newly formed Animal Hope & Wellness Foundation, which funded his rescue operation. Soon after, he developed a line of formulated supplements. Today, Marc runs five businesses, all in the field of healthcare, which includes his free healing practice for animals. He was able to move the shelter to its own space where it can accommodate as many as twenty dogs at a time.

The rescue operation started with one dog. "His name was Gingko and he had been badly beaten. A client told me about him. When I picked him up, he was bleeding badly. I used all my healing skills to fix this dog, and we ended up keeping him. A month later, I got another call. Somebody had heard about a dog who was about to be put down. The vet called, asking me, 'Hey, Marc. Do you think you'd want to help this dog?' And I said, 'Sure.' Then it just started piling up, and suddenly we were getting calls from Animal Control, shelters, and vets about cruelty and abuse situations.

"We started a victim adoption program for dogs and cats. Once they were healed, we would adopt them out, for instance to a rape victim, someone who has suffered through a severe ordeal like the animal has. Together, they would inspire each other to live."

Those are Marc's day jobs. His other mission begins at night. Every few months, he packs two bags, straps on his backpack, and heads to the airport. A kind of Batman for the animal kingdom.

It started in June of 2015, when Marc read about the Yulin Dog Meat Festival, a ten-day celebration of eating dogs, during which an estimated 10,000 dogs are slaughtered to feed festival goers. "Part of me thought it couldn't be true," he says. He knew dogs were eaten in China and other Asian countries—even in America —but he thought the claims of how they were killed must surely be exaggerated. The story went on to explain a widely held belief: that the terror and pain experienced by the dogs—and cats as well—causes their adrenalin to flow, which makes the meat more tender, providing health benefits and enhanced virility. Good luck for the consumer was believed to be another bonus.

Marc was incredulous. He had to see for himself. Over his wife's initial objections—the fact that Marc didn't speak the language and had no contacts there—he flew alone to Beijing and from there to Yulin.

What he saw there, the horror of the brutality he witnessed, changed his life forever. "It was like a war zone; my mind and body went into overdrive. I couldn't think of anything else." He knew he could not rest until he did whatever he could to rescue as many dogs as was humanly possible. Hiring a driver and a translator, and posing as a meat buyer from America interested in importing meat, he was permitted inside the slaughterhouse. Then, using his cell phone, he secretly videoed the killings.

On that first trip, Marc managed to rescue twenty-three dogs; those healthy enough to endure the travel would be brought to shelters in the U.S., including his own. Others were taken to a safe house, to the International Center for Veterinary Services in Beijing, that receives rescues.

When he got home, Marc was so shaken by what he'd seen that it took him days before he could bring himself to talk about it. "I felt I had died inside." With trembling hands, he scrolled through the hundreds of shocking videos and photos he'd managed to take to show to those who were willing to look.

When Marc learned that, according to Humane Society International, thirty million dogs are slaughtered for meat each year to supply the rampant dog meat industry, there was no stopping him. Over the next six months, Marc would make solo trips to Cambodia, Laos, the Philippines, Vietnam, and South Korea. "I thought if I could document the truth of what happens in these places that people don't see, maybe our government will do something about it."

In his journal, Marc wrote about his trip to China: "I left America without a plan. I left America without knowing anyone here. Without making hotel reservations. Without anything but a bag and a ticket. People kept asking me what I came for. I told them it was to save dogs. I told them it was to make whatever change I could with these hands. I spoke about a movement, a belief, and a culture that imbues humanity with compassion. Almost everyone I spoke to held this same belief. Almost everyone I met selflessly extended their hand to me.

"And today, after saving even more dogs and heading off to see a Chinese puppy mill—I found myself surrounded by orphaned Chinese babies and abandoned children. It was here that I found the greatest gift of my journey, a way to make this movement last.

"I will be teaming up with the Little Flower Orphanage to create a more sustained system. They have a farm that I will use to create the first dog sanctuary in Beijing, so that we can save as many dogs as we can from a life of abuse and torture in China. In return, I will pay the orphans there to take care of the dogs. They'll train them and nurture them so they are healthy enough to be adopted out locally, with the more seriously damaged cases being flown back home to Los Angeles to the Animal Hope and Wellness Foundation.

"My hope is that the sanctuary will grow, and that this one starting point will blossom and become many. This is how we'll teach and show the Chinese people how great and amazing dogs are. How they have souls, how they feel pain, how they cry, but most important, how dogs love us no matter what. And they never pass judgement. Regardless of how hard the world may seem, when I come home after a long day, my dog Ginkgo always sleeps under the covers with me. Always continues just to love me.

"You cannot tell a country that does not have the same value system as we to love dogs. The only way is to plant a seed, and to let the dogs themselves soften their hearts. In time, I am certain we will no longer have a society that kills them. Because their lives will now hold meaning.

"I had a lot of opposition coming here—people believing that to risk my life for a single mission did not warrant the sacrifice. But I came anyway. I came because, to me, it was about a movement. It was about saving as many dogs as I could. Or creating something that would last beyond this effort. In the end, it is truly amazing how the world works. How, if our hearts and intentions are pure, it all just seem to come together."

As he writes in his journal, *"Some people are born to be artists or musicians or teachers. I believe I was born to do what I do. Some people find themselves through helping others, the more they rescue, the more they piece themselves back together."*

❧

Marc worked out a routine for his Asian trips. After checking in to his hotel—usually late at night—and putting his passport and cash in the hotel safe, he packs his backpack with a change of clothes (the jeans and T-shirt he's wearing will be covered in blood and dumped at the end of the day) and grabs a few hours' sleep. At dawn, he is picked up by a driver and translator and they head out of the city, stopping along the way for supplies: rope, scissors, flashlights, power cord, wire-cutter, sanitizer, water, extra batteries. Their destination is usually two to three hours out of the city to a rural area where the slaughterhouses are located. Then they wait and watch.

Women with young children from a neighboring village come to watch as trucks, stacked end to end with cages crammed with frightened, whimpering dogs, roll up. Most are stolen pets and guard dogs; some are abandoned street dogs rounded up to sell to meat traders. Children look on as the cages are unloaded onto dollies and wheeled into an abandoned structure used now as a slaughterhouse.

Marc's translator gets out of the truck first and approaches the boss of the operation. He explains he has a rich American businessman with him who's interested in the exportation of dog meat to the States. At a signal from the translator, Marc steps out of the car, cell phone concealed in the crook of his arm, and begins to secretly film. An undercover angel stepping into the darkness to shine a light, risking his life to document the atrocities. More than once, he's been attacked and beaten, a few times badly enough to land him in the hospital. It did not stop him.

He rescues as many dogs as he can and takes them to a prearranged veterinary clinic. Those animals well enough to travel are shipped home to L.A. with him. As of November 2016, Marc had made nine trips to Asia, rescuing more than 1,600 dogs and amassing approximately 5,000 photos and as many videos.

❧

I rescued all the dogs I could, all that were strong enough to survive transport. Saved three cats, and released a pair of rabbits down by a river. Those who died there, I pressed my lips to their skin and shed tears, hoping that even in the darkness, they knew they were not alone.

❧

Through a team of fellow activists, Marc arranged to broker a deal to buy a slaughterhouse in Cambodia, and after getting the dogs out of there, destroy the whole operation. Together, they dismantled the slaughterhouse, pulling up floorboards and tearing down walls until all that was left was a roof and supporting beams, which neighboring villagers pulled to the ground. In exchange, Marc is helping the slaughterhouse owners to make a new start. He and his volunteers are finding them a new location, where they can open a vegetarian noodle restaurant, and are paying their first six months' rent and utilities. "This has taught me a whole lot about compassion and given me new hope for humanity."

Enlisting the help of celebrities Matt Damon, Joaquin Phoenix, and Rooney Mara (among others), as well as veterinarians, activists from America, the UK, Indonesia, and Hong Kong, they have also managed to shut down operations in Korea and Cambodia, rescuing over 200 dogs. "I want the people in China to see that change is possible. People are meeting from all over the world, even within China, to come help us. Our goal is to bring sweeping reform to those countries that permit dog meat trade, and to pass new animal cruelty and protection laws."

❦

In August of 2016, the U.S. Congress invited Marc to speak. He laid out his evidence, and showed what he had filmed. The

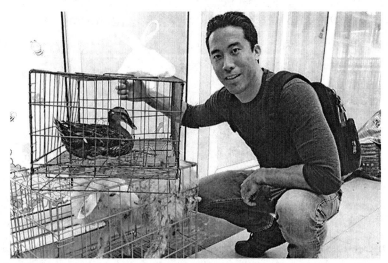

Because all life matters, I rescue ducks, cats, pigs, sheep and chickens from the slaughterhouses whenever I can.

MARC CHING

reaction was outrage. In January of 2017, Marc and his group will sponsor the first federal bill to make the consuming of dog and cat meat illegal in the U.S. His main ally is Representative Alcee Hastings of Florida, who is co-sponsoring the bill.

"When I die, I want to die knowing that I was the best person I could possibly be. That I did what I could with the hands I have and the time I have here on earth, I breathed life into those who could no longer breathe for themselves."

EPILOGUE

$\mathcal{I}$t has been two-and-a-half years since I set out to explore the world of animal healers. I wanted to put to rest the question some critics raised following the publication of my books on healers of people: Could many of the reported healings be ascribed to the placebo response? Placebo, from the Latin, *I shall please*, points to the brain's role in medical treatment. Whether it's the doctor the patient wants to please or the patient's belief system the doctor wants to reinforce or the medicine itself. Sugar pill or protocol, the placebo response has played an important role in medicine for more than two hundred years. So, to some degree those critics were right, there is that element in all healing.

If one believes as I did and do still that all illness and all healing has an emotional component, the placebo response is the very essence of the mind-body connection. The Dalai Lama said, "The mind is the body's greatest physician." I would take it a step further: the mind is also the body's pharmacy.

But those books were about people; animals became the new subject of my inquiry. Because, as I wrote in the introduction to this book, animals have no mechanism for belief or disbelief, the placebo response does not apply. So, something else was operating here, something I would come to learn goes straight to the core of healing itself. Miraculous as many of those healings seem to be, to characterize them as miracles is to miss a deeper truth. Like healers who are dedicated to treating humans, the animal healers I met all seem to have a preternatural capacity for empathy and compassion, which combined with the force of an intention creates its own energy. Then there is the X factor: Love. And an uncanny ability to concentrate that love on a subject, human or animal. As James French of the Trust Technique said, "Our message is all about relationship... and sharing unconditional love with each other, not needy love, but an unconditional love for a healing environment."

The research, the interviews, the time it took to think about and write this book changed me forever. Although a lifetime animal lover, I notice I can no longer look at them as I once did. The dog I pass on the street is not just someone's pet; it is a thinking, feeling being on this earth at this time to share the world with us, its human family.

Animals are not here to entertain or be on display or to be used in scientific/medical experiments; nor are they our property. Those who become our pets have entrusted their lives to us and need our most thoughtful care and respect. We give them food and shelter in exchange for their love and companionship.

Healer and teacher Carol Komitor reminds us that, "We are only one small part of the whole of life on this planet: animals are its heart and soul."

ABOUT THE AUTHOR

Sandy Johnson

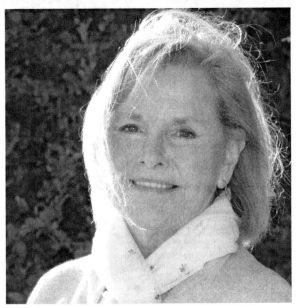

Sandy Johnson lives in Los Angeles with her new puppy, Maddie.

Sandy Johnson, former actress and author of seven previously published fiction and nonfiction books, has traveled to more than forty countries meeting and interviewing spiritual leaders, shamans and healers, including His Holiness the Dalai Lama.

As an actress, Johnson appeared in numerous regional stage productions, and on TV, a running part in *Search for Tomorrow*, as well as guest appearances on various series, and in the feature films *Ash Wednesday* and *Two-Minute Warning*.

In 1979, Johnson published her first novel, *The CUPPI* (Delacorte/Dell), a fictionalized account of a twelve-year-old runaway. The first book to deal with the rising epidemic of teen-aged children taking to the streets, *The CUPPI* (a police acronym for Circumstances Undetermined Pending Police Investigation) was a Literary Guild Selection. Because of the extensive research involving interviews with dozens of runaways, Johnson was called upon to lecture to parent-teacher groups, and law enforcement and social agencies, and made numerous TV appearances: Washington and Philadelphia morning shows, *Good Morning America*, *The Mike Douglas Show*, among them.

As a result of her personal crusade, sections of the book were read into the Congressional Record, and twelve crisis shelters opened in major cities. Stories appeared in newspapers and magazines around the country, including a four-page spread in *People Magazine*. Features ran in *Newsday*, *San Francisco Chronicle*, *Wall Street Journal*, Liz Smith's column, and received rave reviews in *The New York Times*, *Publishers Weekly* and the *Wall Street Journal*. *The Library Journal* featured Johnson's photograph on its cover. *The CUPPI* was published in four languages.

Johnson's second novel, *Walk A Winter Beach* (Delacorte/Dell 1982), was listed on The New York Times Notable Books of the Year list.

In recent years, Johnson's work with Native Americans produced *The Book of Elders: The Life Stories & Wisdom of Great American Indians* (HarperSanFrancisco 1994) and with Tibetans for *The Book of Tibetan Elders*, Introduction written by His Holiness the Dalai Lama (Riverhead 1996).

In 2015, Sandy released *Miracle Dogs: Adventures on Wheels*, which tells the stories of dogs who have gained mobility from the use of "dog wheelchairs."

ACKNOWLEDGEMENTS

My own personal hero, Mark Robinson (and full disclosure: my son) is the founder and inventor of the adjustable wheelchair for dogs, president of Walkin' Pets by HandicappedPets.com, and the Handicapped Pets Foundation. The foundation donates wheels to injured or elderly dogs and other animals that might otherwise be abandoned or put down (see Chris P. Bacon and Emma the baby goat, a miniature pony, and even a bunny rabbit on the HandicappedPets. com website... What's next, wheels for fish?). Mark's company also offers scholarships for veterinarian schools and vet rehab programs. It was clear from an early age that Mark was put on this earth to fix all things or creatures broken; it should come as no great surprise that saving the lives of animals every day became his life's work. Thanks to him this book found its way to print.

Apart from the contributors who so kindly agreed to grace these pages with their remarkable stories, I am grateful to those whose encouragement and support for the project were invaluable: as always and above all, my family, with special thanks to grandsons ten and eleven at the time, Danny Johnson for his vigilant coyote watch on our evening Charley-walks; and Billy Johnson for inspiring *Oopsy Doodle*. My stepdaughter, Debbie Johnson, who read and reread pages was and remains my sunshine.

I am indebted to Teri Rider, publisher, cover artist and editor for her patience and wisdom; Jo-Anne Langstreth for editing; Chris Runge for her superhuman care of Charley and for her help in the search for healers; Masha Nordbye for her abiding support and friendship; Sue Terry for endless readings and editorial suggestions; Kathleen Osman for her tireless transcribing, and to Sam Miller for finding her; Julie Adams for her enduring love and good cheer; Jan Kellar and his mighty semi-colon he tossed my way; Ingrid Watson, champion of the cause.

I am grateful to Dr. Joyce Quan and the people at Glendale Small Animal Hospital for their skillful care; Meredith McHugh for keeping Charley beautiful; Ruthie Steinfeld for keeping my body in working order; and to Marie Anne-Boularand for keeping my soul intact.

And speaking of souls, I will always remember my dear late soul-friend, Alex Street, whose love for animals remains an inspiration.

❧ ❧ ❧

Where to Find our Healers

*M*any of the healers featured in this book have their own practices, have written books, and offer classes in their fields of expertise. Please visit their websites to learn more about these compassionate and dedicated individuals.

Karen Becker, DVM

As a young girl, Karen trained with a Native American shaman who set her on her course. Apart from working in the animal hospital she founded, Karen also founded the Covenant Wildlife Rehabilitation Center, Feathers Bird Clinic, and Therapaw Rehab and Pain Management Center. Thousands of pets dealing with chronic degenerative diseases including allergies, cancer, organ failure, arthritis and auto immune diseases have benefitted from Dr. Becker's unique approach to medicine. Her holistic approach and her passion for clinical pathology (tracking disease processes in the body), as well as an array of integrative diagnostics and innovative treatment protocols have earned her recognition as one of Chicago's Top Vets (according to *Chicago Magazine*), and a special place in her client's hearts.

http://www.drkarenbecker.com/

Anna Breytenbach, Interspecies Communicator, Activist

Anna Breytenbach is a world famous South African interspecies communicator, animal activist, conservationist, and public speaker. She works with cheetahs, lions, wolves, baboons and elephants. Her full-length documentary movie, *The Animal Communicator* has been viewed by millions of people. Anna defines what she does as direct mind-to-mind communication, "although it's as much a matter of the heart as the mind."

http://animalspirit.org/
https://www.youtube.com/watch?v = gvwHHMEDdT0

Cindy Brody, Energetic Healer and Communicator

Cindy is the creator of CinergE, an energetic healing modality that can be applied to all living beings. Her purpose is to help animals to feel mentally and physically better through animal communication and energy work. She has combined her training as a Reiki Master and her intuitive skills to help people and their animals understand each other and to deepen their connection. For the past thirty years, Cindy has been teaching people how to help their pets express their feelings so that they can begin to heal.

http://cindybrody.com/

Marc Ching, Holistic Nutritionist, Healer, Activist

Marc Ching is the founder of The Animal Hope and Wellness Foundation (AHWF), a 501(c)3 non-profit organization that is focused solely on rescuing abused and neglected animals, providing full rehabilitation services and, ultimately, working to help find them their fur-ever families. Ching has not only uncovered the harsh realities of animal abuse, but changed the face of animal rescue throughout the world.

After founding AHWF in 2011, as an appendage to his already thriving natural pet food and wellness company, The PetStaurant, Ching expanded the foundation's reach globally, in 2015, to include rescuing dogs from the horrific Asian dog meat trade.

https://animalhopeandwellness.org/

Margrit Coates, Healer, Communicator

Considered one of the world's leading animal healers, Margrit Coates, who lives near Southampton, England, is also a renowned animal communicator. "I am passionate about helping people with their animals, and I offer a unique service in this respect. When I give healing to your animal I link you in that process, so that you too receive healing energy." Margrit teaches the secrets that enable us to communicate intuitively with our animals.

http://www.theanimalhealer.com

Mary Debono, GCFP

A Guild Certified Feldenkrais® Practitioner with a passion for improving the quality of life for animals and people, Mary discovered the healing power that a heartfelt connection with animals can produce. She created Debono Moves℠ as a way for people to use this connection to generate well-being and vitality in both themselves and their animal companions. Useful for all ages and physical conditions, Debono Moves can help animals move more freely, minimize the effects of aging and injury, improve athletic performance and enhance communication and harmony between human and animal.

https://www.debonomoves.com/

James French, Trust Technique Communicator

Manager of the Mane Chance Sanctuary in Sussex, England, James asks, "What would you say if you were told that the key to taking your relationship with your animals to a new level is as simple as clearing your mind of all thoughts, similar to meditation but even quicker and simpler? Or that this technique can offer the breakthrough with animals that are so distressed, for whatever reason, that even approaching them has seemed impossible?" That, in a nutshell, is the principle of the Trust Technique, pioneered by

James French. To practice the Trust Technique one must change one's own mental state to calm and positively influence the behavior of animals. In this way, animals can be seen as 'mirrors' of our own emotional state, highlighting when our own thoughts may be disordered and in need of rebalancing. The Technique works just as well for animals with which one is unfamiliar as it does for beloved pets, making it a highly powerful method for anyone wishing to work with abused and rescued animals.

https://trust-technique.com/

Leslie Gallagher, CCMT, CCRT

Founder and president of Two Hands Four Paws, a rehabilitation center in Santa Monica, California, Leslie's love affair with animals began during childhood on her family's farm. The center's staff consists of veterinarians, acupuncturists, Doctors of Physical Therapy, RVTs, and Certified Canine Rehabilitation Practitioners; a dedicated group of individuals whose passion is helping animals heal through physical rehabilitation. Leslie's mission is to help every dog that walks through her doors lead a happier, pain-free life regardless of age.

http://www.twohandsfourpaws.com/

Anthony P. George, DVM,
Certified Veterinary Acupuncturist

"Tony," a well-known veterinarian in Los Angeles, has been performing acupuncture on pets in their homes for over fourteen years. He traveled with the Chi Institute to attend the first International Conference on Traditional Chinese Veterinary Medicine in Lanzhou, China.

http://www.dranthonygeorge.com/

Eileen Haworth, DC

The first chiropractor invited to join the staff of the United States Olympic Team Medical staff for the 1984 Summer Olympic Games in Los Angeles, Dr. Haworth continued to work with the United States Olympic Organizing Committee for the next seven years. "Because I'm biomechanically oriented, the importance of flexion and extension and full range of motion is of interest to me—as is my interest in biomechanics and movement. Just as family veterinarians are trained to treat internal problems, my main thing is mechanics."

http://www.k9chiro.com/

Carol Komitor, Energy Therapy

Carol Komitor, founder and director of Healing Touch for Animals®, believes her purpose in life is to be a voice for the animals. "Because if they become extinct, we will, too. We are only one small part of the whole of life on this planet; animals are its heart and soul, especially domestic animals. Whether a dog, a cat, a guinea pig, or a goldfish in a bowl that lives on the kitchen counter like mine and does a little dance whenever I walk by, they all come from a place of unconditional love."

https://www.healingtouchforanimals.com/

Kathleen Prasad, Reiki Practitioner

Author, teacher and practitioner, Kathleen teaches classes both at BrightHaven hospice and sanctuary in Northern California and at partner sanctuaries around the world. "My passion is to share Reiki with animals of all species, and to teach people who love animals how to connect more deeply with them. Healing starts where our hearts connect. Reiki offers simple techniques that anyone can do, and that helps us to open our hearts to the animals and the world around us. When we live our lives in this open and present way, animals, who are pure and sensitive, feel it and are drawn to us and want to share with us and support us. A beautiful, peaceful, compassionate space that embraces, connects and encompasses all beings, all species, all life: this is Reiki in action." Kathleen teaches us how to access our intuition to connect to the animals in our lives.

https://www.animalreikisource.com/

Allen M. Schoen, DVM, MS, Ph.D (hon)
Holistic Integrative Veterinarian

A trailblazer in veterinary acupuncture and natural therapies, developing and practicing them since 1981, Allen Schoen has been acknowledged worldwide for introducing the concept of an integrative approach to veterinary medicine and bridging the gap between conventional and alternative medicine. With over 30 years of clinical experience, teaching, and research, he has developed his own unique integrative approach to animal health care.

http://www.drschoen.com/

Elizabeth Whiter, MHAO MNFSH IIZ Dip. WSA,
Holistic Animal Healer

Elizabeth's home and clinic are situated in the South Downs National Park, in Sussex, England. She founded the only organisations in the United Kingdom that offer a two-year healing course for animals and their human guardians as well. Currently, there are four hundred graduates all over the world who have completed her training, and many of her students and graduates join her every year to offer healing and complementary rehabilitation skills at animal charities in the UK, Cyprus, Sri Lanka, Egypt, South Africa and many other parts of Europe.

She describes how her beloved injured horse taught her how to heal him.

http://www.elizabethwhiter.com/

CPSIA information can be obtained
at www.ICGtesting.com
Printed in the USA
FSOW02n1700110917
38643FS